Victory over Cancer"

Science-Based Strategies To Heal And Prevent Recurrence. The Stories Of Survivors Who Used The Holistic Approach

GERVAIS DZUDIE

Dedication

To my father and many others whose journeys ended too soon while fighting cancer, your memory fueled me and continues to guide me. To all who are still fighting this relentless battle in pain and resilience. May this book be a torch of knowledge for you, your family, or caregiver, offering you love, comfort, and clarity in your decision-making.

Acknowledgment

My deepest gratitude goes to my wife, Gaelle, and my four kids: you stood there in the darkest moments, walking beside me through every storm and moment of uncertainty. To the caregivers, doctors, researchers, and brave survivors who shared their stories, especially Louis Smith, for his leadership, you are the heartbeat of this book. Your courage, compassion, and faith remind me that healing is both a science and a journey of the soul.

About the Author

Dr. Gervais Dzudie holds a Master of Science in Petroleum Engineering from Texas A&M University and a Ph.D. in Information Systems. With over two decades of experience as an Engineering Manager and Data Scientist analyzing complex data to optimize performance in global energy companies, he brings the same analytical precision to understanding cancer. After his own battle with an aggressive prostate cancer.

Dr. Dzudie turned his scientific mindset towards evidence-based strategies for survival and recurrence prevention by transforming research findings, clinical data, and lived experiences from survivors into a practical blueprint that empowers patients to overcome cancer and reduce the risk of recurrence.

PREFACE

If you are reading this book, you probably have cancer or are caring for someone who has cancer. Yes, cancer is a very serious, life-threatening condition that often causes fear, anxiety, and hopelessness due to our lack of knowledge. This book, however, is not intended to feed you false hope, but I want to make sure that you know all cancers are treatable and curable at all stages if you take massive action.

I've written this book to educate my readers about surviving cancer, bringing all the vital tools and practical tips that can be utilized right away.

In this book, you will learn the causes of cancer, understand your diagnosis, your prognosis, and will be equipped with enough knowledge and decision-making data that empowers you to choose a therapy. Therapy that can make a difference between you dying prematurely or beating cancer and living life up to your god given longevity, one that is free of cancer.

I wrote this book because I don't want you to be like the majority of cancer patients who are just helpless and powerless victims waiting on the healthcare industry or their doctors to save them.

According to Worldwide cancer incidence statistics (2015), it is estimated that by 2040, there will be 28 million new cases of cancer and 16.2 million deaths worldwide (1). Are these people only dying from the disease or from the treatment? We won't know that if we don't understand what causes the disease. Arguably, the most devastating disease there is on earth, and if we don't target cancer at its roots, it never goes away once it invades and embeds itself within our bodies. Cancer attempts to disrupt our lives, derailing our plan and stealing our dreams.

At some point in our lives, and due to several circumstances that we will explore in this book, our cells will become injured and develop pre-cancerous or cancerous cells. Not all such cells develop into a tumor because our immune system repairs itself by identifying and eliminating bad cells, such as viruses, bacteria, parasites, pathogens, etc. However, when the body is deprived of essential nutrients, bad cells can mutate and divide uncontrollably in order to survive. This staggering finding highlights the urgency of addressing nutritional deficiencies head-on.

Conventional cancer therapies such as surgery, radiation or chemotherapy do not always yield positive outcomes. Moreover, diet and nutritional therapies that are valuable tools in the treatment arsenal are also often ignored despite an emerging body of research and literature published in 2022 by journals such as Cancer Research and the Journal of Nutrition (2), suggesting that nutrition improves cancer treatment outcomes.

Why are oncologists not routinely discussing nutritional interventions with their patients and why are the voices of holistic practitioners and nutritionists drowned out by the dominant narrative of pharmacological solutions?

By not integrating holistic approaches alongside cancer treatment, patients are missing out on life-changing opportunities to nurture their whole body and prevent recurrence. Instead, they focus on eradicating the tumor that can regrow at some point and allow cancer to come back with revenge.

This book is essential for anyone facing cancer for the following reasons:

1. It weaves in compelling real-life stories of survivors, illustrating diverse journeys and approaches to overcoming cancer in a narrative style that makes complex medical concepts more relatable.
2. It goes beyond conventional treatment by integrating holistic strategies, lifestyle changes, nutrition, mental health, and community support, providing a well-rounded perspective on cancer care.
3. Survivors' stories are supported by the latest research and data, offering readers not just hope but also actionable strategies grounded in science. This dual approach empowers readers to make informed decisions about their health.
4. The book includes a structured plan for readers, breaking down steps to prevent recurrence and foster resilience, making it a practical guide that both patients and caregivers can implement right away.

Disclaimer

The information, ideas, and strategies presented in this book are intended for informational purposes only and are not a substitute for professional medical advice, diagnosis, or treatment. The content of this book is based on the author's personal experiences and research, and it is meant to provide readers with insights and suggestions that may complement conventional traditional cancer treatments.

The results shared in this book are not typical; achieving similar results requires change and massive action. Your efforts, dedication, and the resources you put into the process will dictate your success.

While the supplements and nutritional plans suggested in this book can be helpful, we cannot guarantee that a specific dosage or recommendation is the solution for any particular diagnosis. We strongly encourage patients to take an active role in their treatment, using this information as a starting point for discussions with their oncologist or healthcare provider. Readers should always consult their physician or health-care professionals who are specialists in their fields before implementing any of the suggestions or making changes to their treatment plans, diet, or exercises.

The author and publisher expressly disclaim any liability for any adverse effects, injuries, or outcomes directly or indirectly resulting from the use or application of the information contained in this book.

Every individual's situation is unique, and any decisions about medical care should be made in consultation with a healthcare professional.

Introduction

The Journey Begins Here

Not too long ago, my life took an unexpected turn when I received a terrifying call from my doctor. At the time, I was in my office discussing a collaborative meeting with my engineering team to execute a project. When my phone rang, I checked my caller ID and realized the number belonged to the local hospital, a number that had never called me before. Sensing the urgency, I excused myself and stepped into the hallway. My urologist's trembling voice echoed through the receiver; a voice I had never heard him use as he usually spoke in a very light-hearted tone.

He said, "Do you have a minute to go over the results of your biopsy?" My heart started racing as I listened to my doctor.

"Unfortunately, it is a very aggressive form of cancer," he said with a heavy heart.

His words hung in the air. I didn't know how to react. At that exact moment, my world had frozen. The doctor gently broke the news as he continued to provide details about my diagnosis, but there was no way to soften the blow of "poor prognosis." I felt my chest tighten with every word he said. Suddenly, I just... stopped hearing him. Like I was underwater, where everything was muffled, and my thoughts were sinking. Under panic, I mistakenly hung up on him, feeling as if the ground had just shifted beneath me.

How did I get here? All these years, all the things I thought I'd have time to do, all my plans, dreams, aspirations, they all seem so meaningless now, yet also like pieces of a life I wanted to live but never really did. Now, I didn't even know if I had the chance to start.

It seemed like a cruel joke; I was angry at life for handing me this. What did I do wrong? I wondered if I missed some signs along the way, moments where I could have changed something, anything, that might have led to a different outcome. It was too late to turn around.

I leaned against the wall, breathing heavily, trying to regain my composure as I faced the whirlwind of fear and uncertainty. The situation was overwhelming, but I knew I had to return to my meeting. I also knew I had to drive down to my doctor's office inthe hope that he would accept an impromptu meeting to discuss the treatment options he was about to propose when I cut him off.

My name is Dr. Gervais Dzudie, a scientist, father of four adorable children, and a devoted husband, and once I was the one receiving that devastating diagnosis. As I took a moment to gather my thoughts, I was reminded of my strengths and the critical role I played in my kids' lives and my extended family.

I also remember that I am a curious researcher with a gift and that giving up to my fate was just not an option.

I returned to my office, forcing a smile as I addressed my engineering team: "I need to be honest with you all, I just received some personal news, and while I am committed to seeing this project through, I have to drive to my doctor's office now." While fear and uncertainty loomed over me, I realized that this diagnosis was not the end, but rather it was a catalyst for a new beginning

Why am I writing this book, and who will benefit from it?

You need inspiration and practical advice if you are fighting cancer or staying with a parent, a child, a sibling, a family member, a friend who lives with cancer or died from it. The journey through Cancer is profoundly transformative, not only for those diagnosed but also for their families and communities. Maybe you are sent or into hospice to die, I want to let you know that fighting Cancer is a challenging but not hopeless battle, as the majority of cancer cases can be cured, and almost all stages are treatable. Losing my father, neighbor, and a dozen friends to Cancer, having been a patient myself, interviewing cancer warriors, and understanding the complexities of each cancer treatment, I want to encourage you to break free from the conventional mindset. I thought our stories, narratives, anecdotes, and testimonies would be relevant in the decision-making of each cancer patient.

As a cancer survivor with a background in organizational learning and deep involvement with academic research, I thought weaving together my lived experience with science insights would be more impactful in offering inspiration and actionable insights to those fighting against this disease.

This book is not just about narrating my personal experience, but it is a culmination of hope, resilience, and simplified scientific knowledge aimed at empowering others and their families facing battles. As an engineer and PhD researcher, I enjoy drilling through sciences to make a complex subject like cancer meaningful to everyone. You don't need to be sophisticated and know the mumbo jumbo of scientific details to understand this material. I break down scientific studies available through the literature to combat cancer. My end goal is to come up with a roadmap, a master plan that merges personal resilience with scientific understanding.

Ultimately, this book is a testament to the human spirit's ability to overcome adversity. It's a call to action for anyone to revisit conventional treatment.

Should you refuse or reject conventional treatments?

Treatment decision-making is a personal ongoing process that requires adequate support, information, and time. My book is not a rejection of conventional treatments like surgery, chemotherapy, or radiation that target the tumor in order to help the patients achieve remission. However, as good as these targeted therapies can help in shrinking or removing the tumor in the beginning, science and experience prove that often they fail to repair the issue at the root cause. Instead, this book discusses various adjuvant treatments to take care of the cellular injuries and deeply rooted imbalances that cause cancer in the first place, so it doesn't come back. It emphasizes the science behind the importance of food and nutrition as a powerful tool in the cancer-fighting toolbox. This critical tool is often overlooked by most doctors and patients. While the cancer-fighting community focuses primarily on traditional approaches, research shows that proper nutrition not only boosts the healing process but, in most cases, contributes to a cure. This book aims to bring attention to this vital aspect, empowering patients to take control of the journey and not let only the doctor decide on their fate.

Embracing the challenge: The power of courage, hope, and faith

When I received my cancer diagnosis, a storm of fear and uncertainty enveloped me. More frightening, the prospect of dying and leaving behind my baby daughter, Britany, at such a young age was unbearable. I wanted to be there to witness her grow, to see her first steps into adulthood, and to support her as she navigates life's joys and challenges. My heart ached at the thought of missing Prince's triumphs on the football field and Patrick's success basketball, celebrating Brianna's graduations, watching her navigate college, seeing my beautiful young wife juggling between her medical career and raising our kids as a widow. I wanted to enjoy every moment with my children and watch them start families of their own. I yearned to be grandfather, to leave behind a legacy filled with love and resilience.

Amid the chaos, I found a spark—a deep-seated belief that I would not go down without a fight. Hope became my anchor, courage my shield, and faith the guiding light that illuminated my path. In those early days, my wife and I kneeled down and prayed and cried at every doctor visit, but instead of viewing this diagnosis as a curse, we chose to see it as an opportunity, a call to reshape our health, to find or renew my purpose, strengthen our connection with ourselves and those dear to us.

Getting a cancer diagnosis should not only trigger your survival instinct; it is about beginning your transformation. It is about recognizing that within every struggle lies a chance to revamp your health, to become closer to your loved ones and renew your spirit. To reflect on what truly matters in your life and what gift you have yet to offer the world. You must make a conscious decision to create a new reality aligned with healing. I started filtering every thought, every emotion, and every action through a positive belief system. I envisioned a future filled with moments I longed to experience, a life intertwined with the people I loved most. I believed that God had a purpose for me, that this challenge was not just a battle but a preparation for a greater mission ahead. All these findings made me realize that cancer doesn't define me, and I had the power to turn my experience into a source of hope not only for me and my family, but for everyone else walking a similar path. I wanted to let my renewed spirit be a testament that even in life's darkest moments, there is always light. It is my hope that my story will inspire you, empower you, and others to face cancer with strength and knowledge. Knowing that they too can emerge from their struggles with a stronger mind, soul, and body completely healed from cancer.

Overview of what lies ahead in the coming chapter

Embark with me on a transformative journey with "Victory Over Cancer ". This comprehensive guide contains 10 chapters:

Chapter 1 begins by demystifying the myriad theories surrounding cancer's origins.

Chapter 2 simplifies the complex science behind the disease with a unifying theory of what causes cancer.

Chapter 3 empowers readers to fully understand their diagnoses, stages, and prognoses.

Chapter 4 discusses how to assemble a robust medical and support team to help you fight cancer.

Chapter 5 provides an in-depth look at conventional treatments and their side effects, preparing readers for the road ahead.

Chapter 6 is the central guide to this book, giving you the master plan for repairing your mitochondria and mindset to beat cancer.

Chapter 7 is enriched with real, inspiring survivor stories that are analyzed through a scientific lens.

Chapter 8 addresses the role and importance of integrative approaches (Holistic cancer treatment).

Chapter 9 offers tips to reprogram your bloodstream after treatment, triggering cancer stem cells to self-destruct and prevent recurrence.

Chapter 10 culminates in a compelling call to action.

As its structure highlights, this book is not just about battling cancer; it's about emerging victorious and living a life free of its shadow. By its structure, this book balances personal inspiration, scientific information, and practical strategies, making the book both relatable and informative.

Contents

Chapter 1:
Understanding Cancer through theories of origin

1.1. Definition of cancer

The body is made up of billion or trillion cells in the brain, the blood, and the guts. Some of these cells are dying and being replaced by new cells at a certain frequency. For example: Red Blood cells live about four months; White Blood cells live on average for about a year; Colon cells live for about only four days; brain cells live for a lifetime. Cancer is a non-communicable disease that starts with only one of the trillion cells start to grow and multiply in an abnormal, uncontrolled way from a specific location, where it forms or may not form a mass called tumor, before spreading to other parts of the body.

We are empowered to choose to live a cancer-preventing lifestyle or a cancer-producing lifestyle. Some of the known preventable causes of cancer are:

- Deficiencies in cellular nutrition (alcohol, sugar does the most damage)
- Environmental agents (pesticides and household products, tobacco, air and water pollution)
- Occupation (X-rays, radiation at airports, electromagnetic frequency)
- Location (Industry, Petroleum, mining, construction)
- Drugs (synthetics, hormone therapy, diabetic meds, blood pressure)
- Chronic inflammations and injuries

In general, we can break down the risk factors contributing to the onset of cancers into three (3) categories:

1. Physical Carcinogens, like radiation exposure or ultraviolet light
2. Chemical Carcinogens like cigarette smoking, alcohol, and asbestos, water-borne contaminants such as arsenic, or food-borne contaminants from the environment
3. Biological Carcinogens, which can come from viruses, bacteria, and parasites.

Throughout the march of science over the years, many theories have illuminated the quest for understanding these contributing factors. In this chapter, we will explore these theories:

1.2. Cancer Theories Through History

Overview of traditional and emerging theories about the root causes, including genetic, environmental, and lifestyle factors

1. The Somatic Mutation Theory

The prevailing paradigm in the research of cancer origins was that cancer is a genetic disease in which the alteration in the genome of the cell triggers DNA mutation and causes cell proliferation. To understand this theory, we must start with the premise that genes are the building blocks of our body. In fact, at birth we all inherit a pair of genes which are copies of those from our parents. One comes from our father and one from our mother. Once received, our pair of genes divides and copies itself until we have enough. Let's think of DNA (Deoxyribonucleic Acid) as a material existing in our cells that plays the role of an operating manual or blueprint for our cells. DNA carries the hereditary information that decides what type our cell is; what it does (function); when to divide; and when to die (self-destruct). For any given reason, the DNA can be deprogrammed or dysfunctional, giving wrong instructions to your genes, causing them to change and act erratically. This is called mutation.

Strongly supported by the observation in leukemia. Hanahan and Weinberg (2000) argue that the Somatic Mutation Theory (SMT) begins with changes in a single cell that passes it to its progeny by generating a clone of malignant cells (3). The somatic mutation proposes that cancer arises from alterations within the cancer genome leading to oncogene activation or tumor suppressor genes inactivation.

It is important to know that we have two classes or types of cancer genes:

1A. Oncogenes

These are the types of mutated genes that drive the uncontrolled growth of cells and cancer development. When they are not mutated, they are referred to as proto-oncogenes, and they play the very important role in cells function and development by regulating divisions. If we are using the classical analogy with a car, oncogenes would be compared to a dysfunctional car accelerator (gases) that stays continuously pressed. Mutation in these genes means cells won't be stopped from constantly growing and divide out of control and DNA won't be repaired which can lead to cancer. Some well-known oncogenes include HER2, RAS and BCR/ABL1.

1B. Tumor suppressor genes

Tumor suppressor genes act like "brakes" on cell growth in our car analogy. They prevent cells from dividing uncontrollably, ensuring that abnormal cells die or are eliminated. When they are not mutated, they inhibit the tumorigenesis or uncontrolled cell growth and also repair DNA. Some well-known tumor-suppressor genes include P53 that play a key role

in apoptosis (cell dead) and BRCA1 and BRCA2, involved in DNA repair and often mutated in breast and ovarian cancers

The Stem Cell Theory

This theory contends the existence of a subclass of neoplastic cells within a cancer tumor called stem cells (CSC). Supposedly, we have a type of cell in the human body called stem cells that are very slow cycling and normally designed to help repair and regenerate damaged tissues. Just like healthy cells, cancer cells also possess a small subset of cells known as cancer stem cells (CSC). The stem cell theory suggests that cancers are initiated when a small subset of cells, when subjected to genetic or epigenetic events, start to mutate, giving rise to aberrant cells, according to Jordan and Guzman (2006). This small percentage of the total cancer cell population is responsible for patient relapse and metastasis due to their particular ability to resist and survive conventional chemotherapy and radiation (4). In a breast cancer study conducted by Dontu and All (2003), it was demonstrated that traditional cancer treatments such as chemotherapy and radiation target rapidly dividing cells, often leaving behind CSC (5) because they are very slow-cycling and more resilient. Figure 1 illustrates the cancer stem cell theory of tumor development and how relapse initiates after treatment (6). Imagine cancer stem cells as the master seeds of a weed. If you chop the visible part of the weed, the seeds remain in the soil waiting for favorable conditions to sprout again.

CSCs are programmed to evade therapy, they have adapted and learned to survive previous treatments they divide and repopulate, becoming the root source of metastasis. We need to eradicate CSS and create an environment hostile to their growth for a chance to achieve long-term survival.

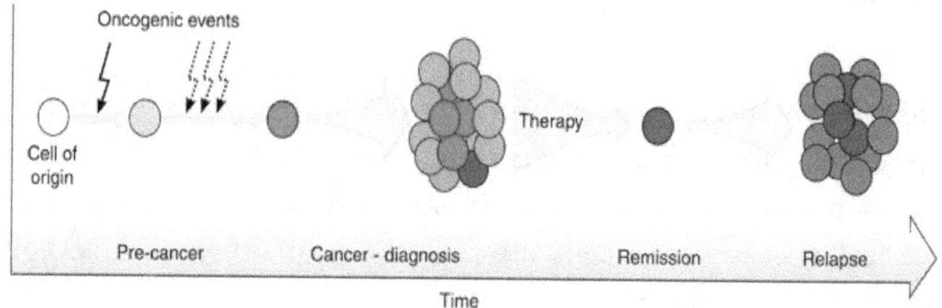

Figure 1. Understanding the cancer stem cell. *Br J Cancer* **103**, 439–445 (2010).

The Parasitology or Bacteria Theory

The human gut microorganisms have a symbiotic relationship with our immunity and capacity to defend against pathogenic invasion. Parasites, when present in the body, eat up the good nutrients and spit out excess lactic acid and other toxic wastes in our body. This contributes to a more acidic environment known to suppress immune function, promoting chronic inflammation and DNA damage. Dr Warren, J. Collin (1891) in his paper: the parasitic Origin of Cancer (7), indicated that cancer might be caused by parasitic organisms that invade and damage body tissues. This is probably why Hippocrates said, "Death sits in the bowls."

In recent years, a provocative hypothesis has emerged from the field of parasitology, suggesting that cancer cells may be akin to intracellular parasites due to striking morphological similarities observed under the microscope. The parasitic theory of cancer posits that cancer cells behave like parasites within the body, infiltrating healthy tissues to use resources and, in doing so, hijacking the immune system to survive and proliferate.

Parasites: Certain parasites like Schistosoma haematobium and Opisthorchis viverrine have been classified as carcinogenic due to their ability to cause long-term infections that trigger chronic inflammation, damage tissue, and create a pro-cancerous environment.

Bacteria and the Microbiome: All the different epithelial barriers of the human body harbor microorganism, from the skin to the respiratory tract to the genital tract to the gastrointestinal tract. Wang et al (2017) argued that the human gut microbiota is a vital organ that carries about 150 times more genes than into the entire body and plays key role in all biological process directly associated with health or diseases (8). Metabolomics and metagenomics studies (9) have demonstrated the dual role of gut microbiota in cancer risk reduction and tumor growth, and anti-cancer therapies (Bultman, 2014). While the microbiome plays an essential role in digestion, immunity, and the absorption of nutrients, research (10) suggests that imbalances within the system that can be caused by disruption of the intestinal ecology (dysbiosis) or exposure to antibiotic can compromises immune fitness, leading to cancer. Backher and Roswall (2015). According to Roy and Trinchieri (2017), the abundant microbiota that is present on the gastrointestinal mucosa and its products and metabolites affect mucosal homeostasis, functions, and immunity (11). A healthy microbiome protects the intestinal lining, keeps inflammation in check, and balances immune responses. When disrupted, however, some bacteria produce metabolites that can be toxic to normal cells, which promotes chronic inflammation, damages the cells, and causes DNA mutation.

The Chemical Theory

This theory of cancer is centered around the role of chemical exposure or toxic substances in initiating mutations and other cellular changes that lead to cancer. It focuses on how carcinogens such as tobacco smoke, asbestos, and certain chemicals induce DNA damage, causing cells to grow uncontrollably. The link between environmental exposure and cancer was published by the English physician and surgeon Percival Pott in 1975.

Pott observed an increased incidence of scrotal cancer in patients who were exposed to soot and coal tar while working as chimney sweepers when they were younger. Brown and Thornton (1957) researched on the topic following such observation between 1714-1788 and found out that these young workers chronically exposed to high level of soot and tartar developed cancer after a long latency (12). This led Yamagiwa and Ichikawa (1918) to develop the first animal cancer model showing causal relationship between chemical exposure and cancer by painting rabbit skin with coal tar to induce tumors (13). In a series of classic experiments, mice were exposed to a single mutagenic chemical (tumor promoter) that led to the initiation of DNA damage by inflammation. However, Takigawa et al (1983) noted that the tumor only grew after multiple repeated exposures (14). Many other reports followed, establishing a link of direct causality between the exposure to various physical and chemical agents and an increased proclivity of developing cancers. For example: Krankheiten and Hirschwald (1894) studied the association between sunlight and skin cancer (15); Harting & Hesse (1979) reported the association between uranium mining and lung cancer (16); as reported by Dietrich and Klaus (2012), Ludwig Rehn studied the association between aniline dye production and bladder cancer in aniline dye workers (17). Ionizing radiation displays electrons from atoms; they can be electromagnetic, such as X-rays used in medical diagnostic CT, or for scanning at the airport, and Gamma rays. It is very clear from epidemiologic studies of radiation workers and Chernobyl atomic bomb victims that ionizing radiation can induce cancer. Mobile phones emit Radiofrequency Radiation (RFR) and generate Electromagnetic Frequency (EMF) potentially linked to malignant tumors in the temporal lobe. Accordingly, a recent study of brain cancer incidents by Frank de Vocht (2016) in the UK suggested that 35% of all cancers recorded between 1985 and 2014 are attributed to mobile phone use (18). Other cases, such as the naturally occurring silicate mineral ASBESTOS, have been clearly linked to DNA damage induction and the development of Mesothelioma.

As demonstrated above, harmful chemicals trigger the production of reactive oxygen species (ROS), damaging cell components including DNA, proteins, and membranes. Other known as mutagens can bind to DNA and cause mutations, chemicals like endocrine disruptors interfere with hormone function, which can promote cell proliferation in tissues sensitive to hormones, such as breast and prostate, increasing cancer risk. This is because DNA is the instruction manual for our cells, and when aggravated by chemicals, it can cause the cells to start acting abnormally, leading to uncontrolled cell growth and division called cancer.

The Nutritional Deficiency Theory

Some elements present in low concentrations in the human body are crucial for a wide range of physiological functions. The nutritional deficiency theory of cancer suggests that an imbalance or a shortage of these key micronutrients can contribute to the development, progression, or recurrence of cancer. The proponents of this theory contend that cancer is not caused by a bacterium, virus, or mysterious toxins, but by the absence of essential nutrients, vitamins or mineral that modern man has removed from his diet. Evidences indicate that the human body needs these food substances to function properly, and their deficiency can cause DNA damage, leading to cancer. According to Campbell (2017), there is a connection of food nutrition and cancer (19), considering that cancer results from an interplay between internal and environment cancer-causing agent with nutrients being the environmental factor. That is why the nutrition theory contends that long-term nutritional deficiencies can weaken the immune system, disrupt cellular function, causing cancer.

In a research paper published in the medical journal in 1968, Indian researchers conducted a study that revealed that when given to rats, aflatoxin produced liver cancer only to rats that were fed with high level protein. By replicating this study, Campbell (19) proved that animal proteins, but not plant proteins were the single most important trigger for turning cancer on and off, like a switch. Furthermore, the cancer-producing effect of highly carcinogenic chemicals were rendered insignificant by a low-protein diet.

The deficiency theory triggered a clear revolution into the sciences and politics of cancer, as they imply that the cure and prevention of cancer can be found in inexpensive food factors rather than in costly research laboratories aiming at proving a therapy. We must be mindful that FDA established protocols to test and evaluate a therapy for approval are so resource-demanding, costly and time-consuming that it can only be played by big pharma. Imagine what reward any company on earth would be able to obtain by spending that kind of money and effort to obtain FDA approval on a food or substances found in nature. This company will never recover its investment because any competitor will now market the product as a substance found in nature, which cannot be patented. The relationship of vitamins and mineral deficiencies and cancer is complex, as research shows that considerable metabolic damage can occur when certain nutrient intake falls below a threshold called the recommended daily allowance (RDA).

Vitamin B17:

Working in a laboratory in 1920's, a San Francisco general practitioner named Dr. Ernst Krebs found that an extract of apricot seeds (referred to as amygdalin, laetrile, or vitamin B17) reduced rodent tumors. The National Institutes of Health Physicians invoke the fact that Laetrile is toxic to cancer cells, most likely because it metabolizes into cyanide, but not other cells, because they have higher levels of beta-glucuronidase enzymes and are deficient in rhodanese enzymes. This suggested the idea that cancer is primarily caused by a deficiency of the vital nutrient (amygdalin) found in the seeds of fruits like apricots, cherries, and apples.

This also justifies that many cultures with low or no cancer rates, like the Humza people of the Himalayas, are attributed to their high intake of apricot seeds.

Vitamin D:

Multiple other studies have shown that low levels of vitamin D3 are associated with an increased risk of various cancers. A study conducted by Creighton University School of Medicine involving 1800 participants proved that supplementation of calcium and vitamin D, especially D3, reduces cancer rate by 77%. Many other retrospective case studies demonstrated that people with most cancers, when evaluated, reported a deficiency in vitamin D. Although we cannot specifically say Vitamin D will cure cancer, there is evidence suggesting a direct correlation between reduced risk of cancer and people with adequate levels of these vitamins is because of the following reasons:

Vitamin D3 controls angiogenesis (regulating cell growth and differentiation), which slows down metastasis by preventing the tumor cell from making new blood supplies.

Vitamin K2 regulates apoptosis (recognizing bad cells and programming their death) versus letting a bad cell stay and multiply by producing a tumor.

Vitamin C:

High-dose vitamin C has garnered significant attention for its potential to enhance the efficacy of immune checkpoint inhibitors, a class of therapies that have revolutionized cancer treatment. Research suggests that vitamin C can play a crucial role in reducing immunosuppression within the tumor microenvironment, which is vital for overcoming the mechanisms that allow tumors to evade the immune system. One of the key benefits of high-dose vitamin C is its ability to promote the infiltration of immune cells, particularly T lymphocytes and natural killer (NK) cells, into the tumor. By facilitating this infiltration, vitamin C enhances the activation of T cells against tumor cells, bolstering the body's immune response. This process is crucial, as a robust immune infiltration can lead to better outcomes in patients receiving immunotherapy.

Moreover, vitamin C enhances intercellular communication within the immune system through the modulation of cytokine production. Cytokines are signaling molecules that play a pivotal role in regulating immune responses, and by promoting their release, high-dose vitamin C can improve the coordination and effectiveness of the immune system in targeting cancer cells. Additionally, vitamin C functions as both an antioxidant and a pro-oxidant, providing a dual action that helps protect against oxidative stress, which is often elevated in cancerous tissues. This balance can create a more favorable environment for immune cells to function optimally while also exerting direct cytotoxic effects on tumor cells. Importantly, vitamin C has also been shown to act as a DE methylator of DNA. By altering the methylation patterns of genes associated with tumor growth and immune evasion, high-dose vitamin C may help reactivate tumor suppressor genes, further enhancing the immune system's ability to recognize and destroy cancer cells.

In summary, the integration of high-dose vitamin C into cancer treatment regimens, particularly in conjunction with immune checkpoint inhibitors, represents a promising approach to not only enhance therapeutic efficacy but also to reinvigorate the body's immune defenses against cancer. As research continues, the potential of this vitamin as a supportive therapy in oncology will likely become more defined, offering hope for improved patient outcomes.

Zinc:

Zinc is the most abundant trace element there is and can be obtained from the diet. When zinc is taken up in the intestine, it is distributed to various target organs where it plays an essential role in DNA synthesis and repair, Immune function (especially T-cell activity), Antioxidant enzymatic activity, Apoptosis (programmed cell death), protein folding, and maintaining the integrity of the p53 tumor suppressor gene. When zinc is at a very low level, the body loses a key protection ability against DNA damage and immune surveillance. In recent years, multiple meta-analyses and reviews have looked into the link between low levels of zinc and many types of cancer. For example, a healthy prostate tissue contains high zinc levels, but in prostate cancer cells, zinc levels are reduced. Hence, zinc level measurement can be used as a diagnostic biomarker for cancer and is ultimately a useful clinical tool for predicting outcomes and even treating patients with cancer. A 2022 review by Venturelli et al explored the associations between cancer and minerals and trace elements (20). Studies show that reintroducing zinc to prostate cancer cells in vitro can inhibit their proliferation. **Prasad et al (1961)** were pioneers in linking zinc deficiency to impaired metabolism, cellular regulation, poor immune responses, and cancer vulnerability. Restoring zinc helps restore balance metabolically, immunologically, and genetically.

The Metabolic Theory

Emerging evidences now indicate that impaired cellular energy metabolism is a defining characteristic of nearly all cancers. The metabolic theory was pioneered by Dr. otto Warburg's work (1956), who established that tumor cells exhibit altered metabolism, meaning they have damaged respiration (22 and 23). Dr. Warburg discovered that cancer cells prefer to continue fermenting glucose even when oxygen is present (Warburg effect). This is in massive contradiction to Louis Pasteur's observations

(Pasteur Effect), who saw in yeast the ability of cells to stop fermenting glucose and to switch to aerobic respiration in the presence of oxygen. These cancer cells suck down so much glucose and produce large amounts of lactic acid and even today, this phenomenon is confirmed over and over today with radiotracers lighting up on PET SCANS, which indicates areas of high glucose metabolic activities, with a commonly used radiotracer being fluorodeoxyglucose (FDG). The reason cancer cells have to ferment and continue making lactic acid even in a 100% oxygen saturated environment is because they cannot respire. They cannot respire because they have defective respiration apparatus. These findings were published in 2012 in an academic book called "Cancer as a metabolic disease." For many years, Dr. Thomas Seyfried took over and has been championing Warburg's idea with multiple lines of evidence in rebuttal of what was known as the Somatic theory of cancer. Dr. Seyfried slaps across the face the notion that genetic mutation is a primary driver of cancer. He objected by proving that in some cases of cancer, there is dysregulated cells growth but do not have any gene mutation. According to the metabolic theory, unlike healthy cells that use oxygen to produce energy from an oxygen-based respiration process called "oxidative phosphorylation," cancer cells often rely on an alternative method called "aerobic glycolysis," also known as the Warburg effect. This means they strive in oxygen-free environment, preferring to ferment glucose to produce energy even when oxygen is present. This process generates lactic acid as a byproduct, which is dumped into the surrounding tissue, causing an acidic environment. This acidic environment is known to suppress immune function and promote chronic inflammation, which is a risk factor for various cancers, tumor growth, and metastasis. Dr. Seyfried (2012) laid the groundwork of several research studies supporting the idea that aberrant cell metabolism is what causes cancer (24).

The Mold and Mycotoxins Exposure Theory

Mold is a type of fungus that grows and thrives in damp, moist or poorly ventilated environments like basements. It belongs to the kingdom of fungi and can grow on decomposed organic materials. Mold appears fuzzy and can produce spores. We often think of molds as a nuisance that affects the structural integrity of homes, but few realize the potential health risks associated with inhaling these spores over a prolonged time. Molds and fungi found in food and homes produce toxic metabolites called mycotoxins. There are four types of mycotoxins that have been found to be carcinogenic: Aflatoxin; Ochratoxin; Zearalenone and Citrinin Vainio and al (1993) reported that the International Agency for Research on Cancer has run some evaluations on this group of toxins and determined that they are toxic compounds that they are extremely likely to cause cancer in those exposed to them over an extended period of time (25). Noreddine Benkerroum (2019) posits that mycotoxin exposure provides three sources of toxicity that can cause DNA damage in cells, leading to chronic inflammation in the lung and cancers: genotoxicity, acute toxicity, and dysregulation of immune response.

Chapter 2:
Simplifying the Science to a unifying theory of Cancer

In an attempt to understand the presence of cancer, we reviewed several theories that appear to be irreconcilable. Although all are determined to explain the causes of cancer, they did not individually point to a clear-cut path to eradicating cancer. What we know so far is that when a spontaneous cancer is detected, some common factual observations are: abnormal cellular characteristics, and the occurrence of a neoplastic development (abnormal growth) of the cells, driving tumor progression and metastasis. If we are serious about devising an effective therapeutic strategy for the successful treatment of cancer, we must dissect through the complexity of the multitude of hypotheses proposed to understand the biological phenomenon leading to the formation of a cancer cell.

Quick Review of Various Cancer Theories

The genetic lenses or somatic mutation theory of cancer explains that cancer occurs due to the accumulation of a series of mutations within oncogenes and tumor suppressor genes. The alterations of the instructions that control the growth, division, and death of cells result in increased proliferation and decreased cell death.

The deficiency theory of disease suggests that diet can contribute to or cause cancer. According to the theory, cells deprived of essential nutrients such as vitamins and minerals become weakened and vulnerable. As suggested by Vander Heiden and Deberardinis (2017), slowing or stopping the proliferation rate is also equally influenced by nutrient availability (27).

The Cancer Stem Cell theory (CSC) posits that cancer is caused by specific dedifferentiated progenitors known as tumor-initiating cells. According to Reya et al (2011), CSCs possess stem-like features containing diverse cell tumor populations within malignancies and the capacity to self-renew and to seed tumors elsewhere (28)

The metabolic disease viewpoint sees cancer as a breakdown or alteration in cell metabolism, meaning how cells create and use energy. Switching to an inefficient or insufficient respiration process is what causes aerobic fermentation that fuels cancer and its rapid, abnormal growth.

The parasitic or microbial viewpoint suggests that some tiny microbes or organisms originating outside the body can invade us, setting up infections, triggering chronic inflammation, and ultimately damaging the cells, leading to cancer. Some studies favor the microparasitic origins of cancer, such as William Coley's approach of treating cancer with bacterial immunotherapy (Coley's toxin). Coley was treating cancer patients by injecting Streptococcus pyogenes directly into inoperable tumors. This provoked a full-blown infection that raised the patient's temperature, mobilizing the body's immune system (28). In his demonstration, Coley inferred that if bacterial toxins were able to kill cancer, it must be because cancer itself was caused by a microbe.

The Mold toxins, environmental and chemical theories all strongly suggest that harmful substances are introduced into our body that can interfere with cellular health. For example, while many molds are harmless, some produce dangerous mycotoxin byproducts, and just as the environmental and chemical theories, when substances with carcinogenic potential are inhaled, ingested, or in direct contact with our skin, they can weaken our immune system.

Observation of the biological phenomenon leading to cancer

Whether cancer develops after exposure to viruses, bacteria, parasites, dietary substances, other carcinogens, or even a sporadic occurrence where no such exposure is evident, the process of malignant transformation takes time and usually does not become apparent until after many years of progressive changes in tissue structure (Fig. 1). Although cancer genomics reveal the presence of mutations in the cell, they are often inconsistent and appear downstream after severe disruptions. Epigenetics reveals how external conditions or environmental factors can flip genetic switches without altering the DNA code sequence in the nucleus (DNA), but rather echoing a change in (mtDNA) function and how the cell processes energy. Cancer stem cells and metastasis both point to a primitive survival-driven state fueled by profound changes in energy demands.

Bottom line is that all hypotheses and paths converge to a fundamental biological flaw that makes the cell misbehave. Whatever organism or phenomenon or agent causing cancer once it takes hold of a normal cell changes the behavior of that cell, turning it into an anaerobic cell (an anaerobic cell does not burn oxygen like a normal cell, rather it ferments glucose to get energy). There is a broken or dysfunctional system inside the cell that is disrupting how it uses energy. We only exist because we have energy, we have energy only because we have good functioning mitochondria, which ultimately points to the battery of the cells, our cell's powerhouse, identified as mitochondria. Therefore, the metabolic chaos in the mitochondria sounds like a good explanation of the genetic instability, the epigenetic confusion, as well as the stem-like behavior and the relentless spread. In light of the above explanation, cancer can be caused by many factors or conditions, manifested through several expressions, but triggered by a single and unique cause: a metabolic crisis at the cellular level.

This is why Dr. Thomas Seyfried (2012) and many other researchers argue that mitochondrial dysfunctions are the prime mover of all cancers. We will now review the different organelles within the cell in order to understand how metabolic reprogramming causes downstream mutation and epigenetic drifts.

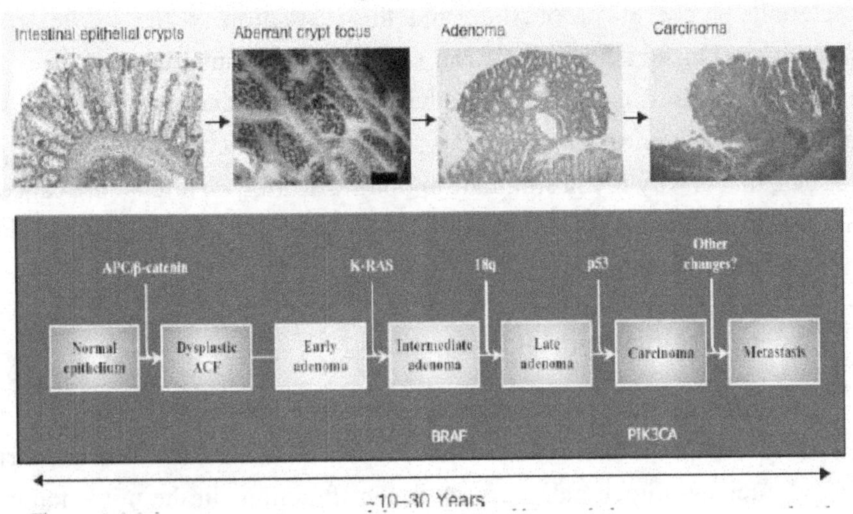

Figure 1. Schematic representation of the genomic and histopathologic steps associated with tumor progression.

Study of main organelles within a cell & understanding of glycolysis & cellular respiration.

In cellular biology, we were taught that there are many internal organs in a cell.

Main organelles within the cell

The nucleus, brain-like central organelle and commanding hub that houses our DNA, which includes the cancer driver genes. Mutations that activate oncogenes or deactivate tumor suppressor genes occur in the DNA within the nucleus. The nucleus also controls gene expression and cell cycle regulation.

The mitochondria (heart). Mitochondria are rod-shaped organelles that constitute the power generators of the cell. Mitochondria also have their own DNA (mtDNA), and mutations in these genes impact metabolism, energy production, and the regulation of the cell's death (apoptosis). In fact, some cells can become dangerous for us; if a cell is not fulfilling its function, it is better to kill it. In cancer, however, the apoptotic program is suppressed, which leads to uncontrolled growth of tissues; that is why if you stimulate apoptotic death, you might cure cancer. To keep the shape and form of our organs, some cells should die, but this must be really balanced.

Nuclear-Mitochondrial interactions

In order to respond to changes in a cell's physiology, there is an ongoing complex interaction between the Nucleus and Mitochondria called nucleus-mitochondria crosstalk. Dysfunctions in the mitochondria will signal the nucleus to alter gene expression, creating feedback that will contribute to cancer advancement.

Glycolysis and cellular respiration

During respiration, mitochondria convert glucose into the biochemical energy Adenosine Triphosphate (ATP) that cells need to survive. There are two types of respiration at the cellular level:

Aerobic respiration (Oxpho)

In aerobic respiration, the cell gets energy when one molecule of glucose from food is broken down in the presence of oxygen gas to produce waste products of carbon dioxide and water. The process is known as Oxidative phosphorylation and releases 32 molecules of ATP.

Anaerobic respiration (Glycolysis)

Studies show that cancer cells prefer anaerobic respiration (fermentation) even in the presence of oxygen. This phenomenon is called glycolysis. During glycolysis, one molecule of glucose is broken down in the absence of oxygen to release only two molecules of ATP, which are used as energy.

Lessons learned and implications for the root causes of cancer

CANCER CELLS USE ENERGY DIFFERENTLY; CANCER CELLS MUST FERMENT. THEY CAN NOT LIVE WITHOUT FERMENTATION BECAUSE THEIR OXPHOS IS INSUFFICIENT.

Whether cancer begins with a mutation, a nutrient deficiency, a metabolic disruption, microbial infection, exposure to radiation, any kind of chemical or toxin, we have shown above that no matter the pathway, something has shifted in the way our cell operates. Therefore, all roads lead to the fact that cancer may be better understood as a metabolic disruption taking root at the cellular level.

The (CYBRID) cytoplasmic hybrid experiment further solidifies the metabolic theory.

We need to first understand cancer epigenetics, which is a branch of science that studies how genes express themselves. It refers to changes in gene expression or cellular function that don't involve alterations to the DNA sequence itself, which means that not every woman with breast cancer genes gets breast cancer, because your diet, lifestyle, behavior, and environment determine whether you will get it or not.

What are known as oncogenic driver genes are present in cancer cells as well as in healthy cells, which means that genes that are implicated in cancer proliferation are ubiquitous. The cybrid experiment is a pivotal study that significantly proves the point that cancer is fundamentally a metabolic disease.

Demonstration and what is a cybrid?

A cybrid (short for *cytoplasmic hybrid*) is a lab-created cell that has:

Nucleus (DNA) from one cell type (often a cancer cell), and Cytoplasm (and mitochondria) from another cell type (usually a normal cell).

This allowed scientists to isolate and test whether nuclear DNA or mitochondrial function is the main driver of cancerous behavior. The researchers posited that if cancer was really caused by a genetic mutation in the nucleus, then inserting a cancerous cell nucleus into a healthy cell should immediately result in a cancer-like behavior. As researchers transferred the nucleus (a section of the cell that houses most of our genes) from a tumor cell and planted it into the fresh cytoplasm of a healthy cell, it still maintained regulated growth and did not become cancerous. However, when the implanted mitochondrial (cytoplasm) came from a cancerous cell, even if the nucleus was from a healthy cell, to their surprise, they noticed dysregulated growth as the cell became immediately cancerous.

Signification: This experiment is proof that cancer arises from a disruption in the mitochondria that generates cellular energy. This supports the metabolic theory, which says: "Cancer is primarily a disease of damaged mitochondrial energy metabolism, and the genetic mutations we see are secondary." In other words, when the cancer cells ferment, mutations collect in the nucleus. If the mitochondria lose their ability to produce energy efficiently, the cell enters its default state, proliferating by fermentation metabolism and consuming large amounts of glucose and amino acids, such as glutamine, to survive. Metabolic regulation is intricately correlated with cancer progression.

Introduction to Angiogenesis and Implications

Tumors require sustenance in the form of nutrients, and seek to evacuate metabolic waste and carbon dioxide, just like normal tissues. As a tumor grows, it reaches a point where it needs more nutrients than nearby blood vessels can provide. The tumor then releases angiogenic factors in the system, such as VEGF (vascular endothelial growth factor), which sprout new blood vessels around existing ones, allowing the tumor to grow larger and spread to other parts of the body. Excessive branching of distorted, enlarged vessels induces erratic blood flow into the system, leading to metastasis. This is why anti-angiogenic therapies allow the blocking of these new blood supplies, starving the tumor to death.

Sources of Fuel:

We can identify some preferred fuel sources and intake pathways that cancer uses to metabolize substances into necessary food for survival. The two key areas are Glucose and Amino acids, mainly Glutamine.

Glucose

Produced from carbohydrates, but can also be produced from proteins.

Higher glucose consumption rates: most cancer cells are addicted to insulin and sugar like 200 times more than normal cells, because they are using the very difficult method "glycolysis" seen above, to turn glucose into energy. Normal cells also use glucose to produce fuel, but they are like our modern hybrid cars; they actually use less glucose to function. However, when necessary, they can switch to the backup energy source called Ketone.

Amino-Acid

While people are familiar with the idea that cancer cells thrive on glucose, not many are aware that amino acids, which are protein's building blocks, are the second most used energy source for cancer cells. Targeting amino acid metabolism is a very challenging and selective task, because the nutrients are vital for the growth of normal cells.

What are some key amino acids that feed cancer cells?

Glutamine: The most significant amino acid in cancer metabolism, acting as a source of nitrogen and carbon. Cancer cells are addicted to glutamine; they use it in a process called glutaminolysis, breaking amino acid glutamine into pathways that fuel rapid growth in very aggressive cancers.

Serine and Glycine: These are non-essential amino acids. They are very important for biosynthetic pathways, for generating materials that cancer needs for division.

Arginine: Another amino acid cancer cells rely on to grow, as it supports the synthesis of polyamines that play a role in cell signaling. Some cancers are arginine auxotrophic, which means they can't produce arginine for themselves and rely on provision from their environment.

Bad food: Nitrites are a potential killer. Nitrites found in processed meat such as bacon, sausage, and hot dogs help to form nitrosamines in the body, which implies that they help to cause cancer.

UNIFYING THEORY AND KEY TAKEAWAY

A carcinogen stemming from our toxic modern living conditions weakens the membrane of our cells and slips inside the normal cell. Once inside, it intercepts and eats all the glucose entering the cell, excreting mycotoxins (a very dangerous and highly acidic hormone/thick slime) and other harmful garbage inside the cell. With the toxin load increasing into the cell, its mitochondria, which are supposed to convert glucose into energy, become unhealthy and can no longer convert energy into ATP as all the glucose is intercepted. At this point, the unhealthy cell creates a protein coating on its wall that continues to attract and steal more and more glucose, blocking oxygen as the ATP level drops. This is defined as anaerobic. At this point, the cell is forced to survive by using fermentation.

Emerging research increasingly supports the view that cancer is fundamentally a metabolic disease rooted in mitochondrial dysfunction. Mitochondria, the cell's energy producers, are crucial for regulating metabolism and apoptosis. When these organelles are impaired, cells may shift to glycolysis for energy production, even in the presence of oxygen, a phenomenon known as the Warburg effect, which facilitates uncontrolled cell proliferation and tumor development.

Several environmental and lifestyle factors contribute to mitochondrial damage, thereby increasing cancer risk. High intake of saturated fats, cholesterol, and processed animal products has been linked to mitochondrial dysfunction and altered lipid metabolism, promoting tumorigenesis. Additionally, exposure to pesticides and herbicides, such as glyphosate found in conventional produce, can induce oxidative stress and impair mitochondrial function.

Lifestyle choices further exacerbate mitochondrial damage. Smoking introduces toxins that harm mitochondrial DNA, while excessive alcohol consumption and high sugar diets contribute to oxidative stress and metabolic imbalance. Physical inactivity and obesity are also associated with reduced mitochondrial efficiency and increased cancer risk.

Recognizing cancer as a metabolic disease underscores the importance of addressing these modifiable risk factors. By adopting healthier diets, reducing exposure to environmental toxins, and engaging in regular physical activity, individuals can support mitochondrial health and potentially reduce their cancer risk.

Implications

Considering the knowledge gained above, metabolic interventions and oxygenation can inhibit tumor growth, altering the entire approach to treating the disease. The proliferation of cancer is correlated with the availability of nutrients. That is why diet and fasting can starve cancer cells, allowing them to repair and restore mitochondrial function. Hence, the path to prevention and healing is one of wholeness, where our cells have the nutrients and support, they just need to repair themselves and stop the tumor growth by taking away the fuel.

Chapter 3: Understanding Your Diagnosis, Staging, and Prognosis

The Pathologist: The hidden hero behind cancer diagnostics

While surgeons remove tumors and oncologists prescribe treatments, pathologists work behind the scenes to unlock the most vital answers about a patient's cancer. A pathologist is a medical doctor who specializes in examining tissues, cells, and bodily fluids to diagnose disease. In cancer care, their work is not just important; it is foundational.

After a biopsy or surgery, the tissue sample is sent to the pathology lab, where the pathologist analyzes it under a microscope. Their job is to determine whether the cells are cancerous, and if so, what type of cancer it is, how aggressive it looks (the grade), and whether it has spread to the surrounding margins. Using special stains and molecular techniques, they may also test for genetic mutations, receptor status (like HER2, estrogen, or progesterone in breast cancer), and biomarkers that guide targeted therapies.

For example, when Fatima, 45, had a lump removed from her breast, her pathologist confirmed it was invasive ductal carcinoma, Grade 2, estrogen receptor positive. This diagnosis directly shaped her treatment, hormone therapy, and a lumpectomy, followed by radiation.

Pathologists also stage the cancer in collaboration with radiologists and oncologists, reviewing lymph node involvement and assessing whether the cancer has invaded blood vessels or lymphatics. Without their report, called the pathology report, no oncologist can proceed confidently with a treatment plan.

In essence, the pathologist provides the biological roadmap of a patient's disease, translating cells into answers that lead to healing. The visual in Figure 2 illustrates the flow from diagnostic to treatment.

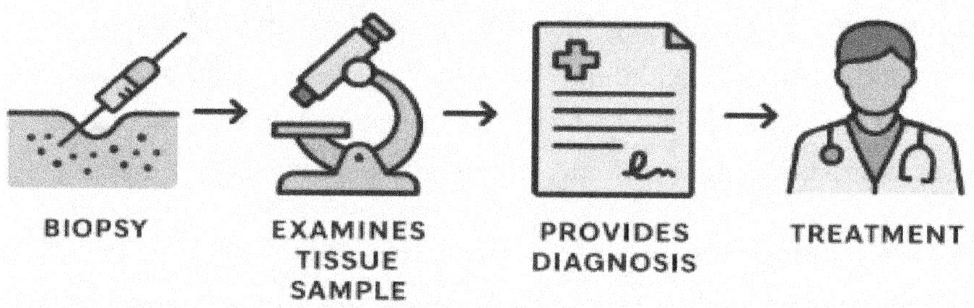

Figure 2. Flow from Biopsy to Treatment

Decoding the diagnostic

Let's assume the pathologist and your doctor, who ordered the diagnostic, have done their job, and you are told that you have cancer. Take the time to fully understand your diagnosis before making a decision. Ask your doctor for a clear explanation of the cancer type, stage, grade, and whether it has spread. Request a copy of your pathology report and review it with a second professional if necessary. Don't hesitate to ask questions, even if they're basic, about unfamiliar terms, treatment options, or the next steps. Consider bringing a trusted friend or loved one to appointments for support and to take notes. Clarity at this stage empowers you to make informed decisions, reduces fear, and helps you develop a treatment plan that aligns with your goals and values. Nowadays, several diagnostic tools are available to provide insights into the presence, location, and behavior of your tumor. These tools range from blood tests to high-resolution imaging, as discussed below:

Tumor Marker Identification. A Blood Clue

When John, a 59-year-old accountant, began feeling increased fatigue and back pain, his doctor ordered a simple blood test. The results showed elevated Prostate-Specific Antigen (PSA) levels, a classic tumor marker associated with prostate cancer. Tumor markers are substances, often proteins, produced by cancer cells or by the body in response to cancer. Others include **CA-125** for ovarian cancer and **CEA** for colorectal cancer. While not definitive alone, they are useful red flags prompting further testing.

Genetic Tumor Markers. The Code Within

Brenda, a 36-year-old woman with a strong family history of breast cancer, opted for genetic screening. She tested positive for a BRCA1 mutation, a hereditary genetic marker that greatly increases the risk of breast and ovarian cancer. Genetic markers, such as BRCA1/2, EGFR, and KRAS, enable doctors to assess inherited risk and personalize treatment plans. In Sarah's case, early detection through genetic screening led to a preventive double mastectomy and peace of mind.

Mammography. Seeing What's Hidden

Every October, during Breast Cancer Awareness Month, Helena scheduled her routine mammogram. This low-dose X-ray of the breast tissue detected a small mass invisible to touch. Fortunately, it was

diagnosed early and successfully treated. Mammography remains the cornerstone of breast cancer screening and has significantly reduced mortality when performed regularly in women over 40.

Magnetic Resonance Imaging (MRI). The Deep Look

Mr. Hardy, a retired teacher, complained of persistent headaches and visual disturbances. A brain **MRI**, using powerful magnets and radio waves, revealed a small glioblastoma. MRI is particularly effective in imaging soft tissue, the brain, spinal cord, and pelvic regions, without exposing the patient to radiation. It provides a sharp contrast between healthy and abnormal tissue.

Computed Tomography (CT) Scan. The Layered Truth

When Mimi, a lifelong smoker, developed a chronic cough and weight loss, her doctor ordered a **CT scan** of the chest. This imaging method uses X-rays to create cross-sectional images of the lungs, and revealed a small nodule in her right lobe. CT scans are invaluable in detecting lung, liver, and pancreatic cancers, as well as assessing the extent to which they have spread.

Fluoroscopy. Motion Picture of the Inside

Andrew, an active 62-year-old, experienced difficulty swallowing. A fluoroscopy with a barium swallow test allowed physicians to observe his esophagus in real-time as he drank a contrast solution. The dynamic images helped identify a narrowing caused by esophageal cancer. Fluoroscopy captures motion inside the body, often used for evaluating the gastrointestinal tract.

Ultrasonography. The Echoes Within

When Alice's doctor palpated a mass in her abdomen, an ultrasound

was the first diagnostic step. The scan, using high-frequency sound waves, revealed a cystic lesion in her liver. Ultrasound is widely used for abdominal, pelvic, and breast evaluations, especially in younger women, and during pregnancy when radiation should be avoided.

Endoscopy. Eyes inside the Body

Idriss, 52, had long ignored blood in his stool until he agreed to a colonoscopy, a form of endoscopy that uses a flexible tube with a camera to examine the colon. The procedure discovered early-stage colorectal cancer, which was removed during the same procedure. Endoscopy is key to diagnosing cancers of the digestive and respiratory tracts, and allows for real-time biopsy.

Understanding what staging means and how it guides the treatment

After a cancer diagnosis, one of the most important steps is understanding the stage and grade of the disease. These two factors help doctors assess the extent to which the cancer has progressed and its potential aggressiveness. This information forms the backbone of treatment planning, prognosis estimation, and even clinical trial design based on the experience and outcome of groups of previous patients with a similar stage. Staging gives healthcare providers a common language to describe how far cancer has spread and how serious it is. It serves several key purposes: guiding treatment decisions and estimating prognostics. For example, a prostate cancer or a breast cancer may be treated with surgery only at Stage 1; meanwhile, Stage 4 will require hormone therapy, chemotherapy, or immunotherapy.

The Four Main Stages of Cancer

Several Cancer staging systems are used worldwide, but the most clinically useful is the TNM system (Tumor, Node, and Metastasis)

developed by the AJCC (American Joint Committee on Cancer) in collaboration with the UICC (Union for International Cancer Control). The TNM evaluates and classifies:

T (Tumor) – Size and extent of the primary tumor

N (Nodes) – Involvement of nearby lymph nodes

M (Metastasis) – Whether the cancer has spread to distant organs

From these components, a **stage number (1 to 4)** is assigned:

Stage 1 – Localized Beginnings

Example: A small tumor confined within the prostate gland (localized prostate cancer).

At this stage, the tumor is still small and has not spread to lymph nodes or distant sites. The cancer is usually highly treatable, and often curable with surgery or localized therapy.

Stage 2 – Local Spread

Example: Early-stage breast cancer that has invaded nearby breast tissue, but not lymph nodes.

The tumor is larger or has begun to invade neighboring tissues, but it has not yet metastasized to the lymph nodes or distant organs. It may still be curable, but it may require a combination of treatments like surgery and radiation.

Stage 3 – Regional Lymph Node Involvement

Example: Colon cancer that has spread to the regional lymph nodes.

This stage indicates a more advanced tumor that has spread to nearby

lymph nodes, the body's filtering stations. The presence of cancer in the lymph nodes often means a higher risk of recurrence, and usually calls for aggressive treatment.

Stage 4 – Distant Spread (Metastatic)

Example: Lung cancer that has metastasized to the brain or bones.

Stage 4 cancer has spread beyond its original site, and the lymph nodes, to distant organs such as the liver, lungs, brain, or bones. Although it's often not curable, many patients can live longer and better with targeted therapies or immunotherapy.

Cancer Grading - How the Cells Look

While staging tells you *how far* the cancer has spread, grading tells you *how abnormal* the cancer cells appear under a microscope, depicting how aggressive it is.

Grade 1–3 (or 4): Degree of Differentiation

Grade 1 (Well-differentiated): Cancer cells look a lot like normal cells. Tend to grow slowly.

Grade 2 (Moderately differentiated): Cells are more abnormal and slightly faster-growing.

Grade 3 (Poorly differentiated): Cells look very different from normal, and often grow or spread quickly.

Grade 4 may be used in some systems for the most undifferentiated tumors.

Pathological Diagnosis (Dx): A pathologist confirms the cancer type and grade by examining tissue samples (biopsies). The biopsy not only confirms the presence of cancer, but also provides clues about how aggressive the tumor might be.

A Real Example of Putting It All Together

After her breast biopsy, 49-year-old Elena learned she had Stage 2, Grade 3 triple-negative breast cancer. The cancer had not yet spread to lymph nodes, but was moderately large, and composed of aggressive-looking cells. This diagnosis meant she needed a combined approach of chemotherapy, surgery, and radiation. Her care team used the stage and grade to map a precise battle plan, and four years later, she remains in remission.

The Prognostic Spectrum: How prognosis is determined and what it means for you

When someone is diagnosed with cancer, one of the first questions they ask is: *"What are my chances?"* This question touches on the prognosis, which is a medical forecast about the likely outcome of your cancer. While no prediction is absolute, modern cancer science has developed robust tools to estimate survival and guide treatment decisions.

What influences a patient's prognosis?

A patient's prognosis can be determined by a combination of factors:

Tumor Type and Location: Some cancers (e.g., basal cell carcinoma) are highly curable, while others (e.g., pancreatic adenocarcinoma) tend to be more aggressive.

Tumor Grade: How abnormal the cancer cells look under the microscope. Low-grade tumors resemble normal cells and grow slowly, while high-grade tumors are more aggressive.

Morphologic Variants: Certain rare cell patterns or subtypes of cancer, such as mucinous carcinoma in breast cancer or sarcomatoid carcinoma in lung cancer, may signal either better or worse outcomes, depending on the type. These features are noted by the pathologist and carry prognostic significance because they affect how the tumor behaves.

Molecular Markers: The presence of specific mutations (e.g., BRCA1 in breast cancer or EGFR in lung cancer) can alter prognosis and determine response to targeted therapies.

Is there a tool that clearly stratifies survival chances?

The combination of factors indicated above is used to build a prognostic model that can be leveraged to generate more individualized predictions. This is where pathology becomes a predictive science. Through careful analysis of the primary tumor (T), regional lymph nodes (N), distant metastasis (M), and histologic grade (G), oncologists can sketch a precise map of a patient's disease and estimate how it might behave.

The T category evaluates the size and extent of the primary tumor. If the tumor cannot be assessed, it's labeled TX; if no tumor is found, it is T0. A small, contained tumor may be T1, showing low-grade invasion into nearby tissues. A larger or more locally invasive tumor may be classified as T2, T3, or T4, with T4 indicating invasion into surrounding structures, such as the chest wall or skin (for instance, in breast cancer).

Next, the N category indicates whether cancer has spread to regional lymph nodes, the body's first line of defense. If the lymph nodes cannot be assessed, it is classified as NX; if none are involved, it is classified as N0. If one to three regional nodes are positive, it's classified as N1. More extensive involvement, such as the presence of four or more lymph nodes, progresses to N2 or N3, indicating a more advanced stage of spread.

The M category addresses whether the cancer has traveled beyond its original site to distant organs. M0 means that no distant metastasis has been found, while M1 confirms distant spread to the bones, liver, brain, or lungs, for example, which significantly affects the prognosis.

Finally, the histologic grade (G) indicates how closely the tumor cells resemble normal, healthy cells. G1 tumors are well-differentiated, slow-growing, and typically less aggressive. G2 are moderately differentiated with intermediate behavior. G3 tumors are poorly differentiated, often rapidly growing, and prone to metastasis. If the grade cannot be assessed, it's labeled GX.

Bringing it all together, imagine this combination:

T2 (tumor invades nearby muscle), N1 (cancer in 2 lymph nodes), M0 (no distant metastasis), G2 (moderately differentiated cells).

This profile indicates a stage II or III cancer, depending on the tumor type, with an intermediate prognosis. It suggests that while the cancer has begun to spread locally, it has not yet reached distant organs. With appropriate treatment, including surgery and systemic therapy, survival can be extended significantly.

In contrast, a profile like:

T4, N3, M1, G3 would reflect advanced, high-grade disease, likely Stage IV, with a poorer prognosis, requiring aggressive multi-modality treatment and consideration of quality-of-life goals.

Understanding these categories gives patients clarity and control. It enables their care team to develop targeted therapies, set clear expectations, and benchmark treatment outcomes across cases. In cancer care, staging is not just labeling; it's navigation.

An Example of a Pathology Report to pull it altogether.

Sample Pathology Report (Breast Biopsy)

Patient Name: Rosalie Jordan
DOB: 07-12-1981
Date of Biopsy: 03-18-2024
Specimen: Left breast mass – core needle biopsy
Clinical History: Palpable 2.5 cm mass in the upper outer quadrant of the left breast

Gross Description:

Four tan-white, soft tissue cores measuring from 0.8 cm to 1.5 cm in length, all submitted for microscopic examination.

Microscopic Description:

The tissue shows invasive nests and cords of atypical epithelial cells within a desmoplastic stroma.

The tumor cells exhibit moderate nuclear pleomorphism and mitotic activity.

No evidence of lymphovascular invasion is seen in this biopsy.

Diagnosis:

Invasive Ductal Carcinoma, Grade 2 (Nottingham Histologic Score 6/9)

Tumor size on biopsy: Cannot be determined from core biopsy

Lymphovascular invasion: Not identified

Estrogen Receptor (ER): Positive (90%)

Progesterone Receptor (PR): Positive (70%)

HER2: Negative (IHC score 1+)

Ki-67 (Proliferation Index): 22%

Comment:

This intermediate-grade, hormone-receptor-positive breast cancer may respond well to endocrine therapy. HER2-negative status suggests HER2-targeted therapy is not indicated. Further surgical excision and staging are recommended.

What does each section mean?

1. Gross Description:

This describes what the pathologist saw with the naked eye before placing tissue under the microscope.

"Tan-white, soft tissue cores" are the pieces of the tumor removed by needle.

The lengths of each sample are documented for record-keeping purposes and to ensure adequacy.

2. Microscopic Description:

Here, the cellular architecture, as seen under a microscope, is described in detail.

"Invasive nests and cords" refer to the cancer cells that have spread beyond the ducts into the surrounding tissue.

"Atypical epithelial cells" refers to abnormal cancerous cells.

"Desmoplastic stroma" is a fibrous tissue that forms in response to tumor invasion.

"Moderate nuclear pleomorphism and mitotic activity" suggests intermediate aggression.

3. Diagnosis:

This is the conclusion, and arguably the most essential part of the discussion.

Invasive Ductal Carcinoma (IDC): The most common type of breast cancer.

Grade 2: Means intermediate aggressiveness, based on cell appearance and mitotic rate.

Nottingham Score: A scoring system evaluating tubule formation, nuclear pleomorphism, and mitotic count (each 1–3 points). Total 6–9 = Grade 2.

4. Receptor Status:

These determine targeted therapy options:

Estrogen Receptor (ER) Positive (90%) – responds to hormone-blocking treatment.

Progesterone Receptor (PR) Positive (70%) – also hormone-sensitive.

HER2 Negative (IHC 1+) – no overexpression of HER2 protein, so HER2-targeted drugs like Herceptin are not used.

5. Ki-67 Index (22%):

A marker of cell proliferation at a moderate rate. Useful in estimating the rate of cancer growth.

6. Comment:

The pathologist summarizes clinical implications:

ER/PR+ tumors usually respond well to hormone therapy.

HER2− status narrows treatment options.

Surgical excision is needed to determine the full extent of the disease and confirm staging.

Chapter 4:
Assembling Your Medical and Support System

4.1. Building Your Medical Team

The moment a cancer diagnosis is confirmed, there is no need to panic. Don't rush into anything out of fear. You need to have the right attitude and start building a strong, coordinated, and effective support team. It is essential that this team be more than just a group of doctors; rather, it should be a collaborative unit for healing and informed decision-making. You will need a multidisciplinary team to help you navigate the process, and this is how to approach it.

Appoint a Trusted Advocate and a Co-navigator

This is someone very close to you who is available and will genuinely stick around for you, much like a spouse, a very loyal family member, or a close friend. This person will do the following:

- Attend appointments with you
- Take notes
- Ask questions on your behalf
- Help manage information overload

Assemble your core medical team.

This includes:

- **Oncologist** – your primary cancer doctor
- **Surgeon** – if surgery is needed

- **Radiation oncologist** – if radiation therapy is part of treatment
- **Pathologist** – who interprets biopsy results
- **Primary care physician** – for overall health and coordination
- **Dietitian** – you need one with oncology experience to help with nutrition during cancer treatment
- **Mental health counselor** – to help process the emotional toll

Ask each provider about their experience with your specific type of cancer and ensure they're comfortable integrating and collaborating with other specialists.

Join a Cancer Support Group

Seek out in-person or online cancer communities and groups that are specific to your type of cancer when possible, as they offer:

- Emotional support
- A judgment-free place to vent
- Reduce isolation
- Practical tips from survivors
- A safe space to vent or ask questions

Cancer support groups or communities are incredibly valuable environments where warriors and long-time survivors are candid about sharing their journeys and personal experiences, reducing fear, anger, and sadness, and providing comfort and a sense of belonging. Besides personal anecdotes, many of these groups share reputable articles and research updates on the disease. However, one must be cautious to avoid misinformation, unverified medical advice, pseudoscience, and harmful myths that are being disseminated in some unmoderated groups.

Some very popular online cancer support options are: Reddit, Facebook groups, Inspire, Cancer Care, and Smart Patients.

4.2 The Importance of Emotional Support Groups: Family, Friends, and Therapy.

No one should withdraw and isolate themselves after a cancer diagnosis. A cancer diagnosis is more than a physical event, and it ripples through every corner of a person's emotional and social life. In this vulnerable period, emotional support becomes not just helpful but potentially lifesaving. The presence of caring family members, close friends, support groups, and available mental health professionals can form a powerful web of resilience around the person diagnosed. These relationships serve as emotional anchors, helping patients cope with fear, uncertainty, and treatment-related stress, while reducing the risk of depression and anxiety.

Scientific evidence has confirmed that no one should walk the cancer journey alone. In a landmark study titled *Postdiagnosis Social Networks and Breast Cancer Mortality in the After Breast Cancer Pooling Project*, Kroenke et al. (2016) found that socially isolated women had a 33% higher risk of breast cancer–specific mortality and a 43% higher risk of overall mortality compared to women with robust social networks (29). The researchers emphasized that post-diagnosis social support, particularly from friends, relatives, and the community, plays a critical role in both psychological well-being and survival outcomes. The findings underscore that having people to lean on is not a luxury; it is a crucial determinant of life and death. Support groups offer a space where patients can share openly without fear of judgment, whether in person or online. This helps them connect with those going through similar experiences, serving to reduce feelings of isolation. Additionally, mental therapy guided by psychologists or psycho-oncologists trained in cancer care can help patients process grief, manage anxiety, and regain a sense of control.

As a survivor, Maya R. recalled, "It wasn't the chemo that broke me; it was the nights I felt alone. What saved me was knowing some people saw me, listened to me, and stood with me."

Therefore, you should reach out, build your circle, and allow yourself to be supported, emotionally, spiritually, and mentally. In doing so, you not only improve your quality of life but also increase your chances of survival. To find a healing support group in your area, please go to: Home, Healing Strong.

Chapter 5:
Understanding Conventional Treatments and Their Side Effects

5.1 Overview of Conventional Treatments: Surgery, chemotherapy, radiation, and immunotherapy.

Surgical Treatment

Surgery remains one of the cornerstone treatments for cancer, especially when the disease is detected at an early stage. The primary goal of cancer surgery is to remove the tumor entirely or, when that's not possible, to excise as much of the cancerous tissue as feasible. This approach not only aims to eliminate the source of the malignancy but also prevents further spread to nearby organs or lymph nodes. The effectiveness of surgical intervention largely depends on the **size**, **type**, and **location** of the tumor. For instance, tumors that are localized and have not yet invaded surrounding tissues or spread to distant organs often offer the best outcomes when surgically removed. A small, well-defined breast tumor may be removed through a lumpectomy, preserving most of the breast. In contrast, a more aggressive or deep-seated pancreatic tumor might require a more extensive operation like a Whipple procedure. Moreover, the possibility of achieving "clean margins," meaning no cancer cells are found at the edges of the removed tissue, is a critical factor in determining surgical success and minimizing recurrence. Ultimately, when performed early and appropriately, surgery can offer a curative outcome or serve as a crucial first step in a comprehensive treatment plan involving chemotherapy or radiation therapy.

Chemotherapy Treatment

Chemotherapy is a cornerstone in cancer treatment, designed to eradicate tumor cells while sparing normal tissue as much as possible. Chemotherapy can be very crude as it targets any cell that divides at a fast rate. Its primary goal is to eliminate cancerous cells throughout the body, including those that may have spread beyond the primary tumor site but are not yet detectable, a concept known as controlling disseminated subclinical disease. This systemic approach is particularly vital for treating elementary lesions and preventing metastasis.

The effectiveness of chemotherapy can vary depending on several factors, including the size and location of the tumor. Smaller tumors with high growth rates often respond better to chemotherapy, as the drugs target rapidly dividing cells. Conversely, larger tumors or those located in areas with limited blood supply may be less accessible to chemotherapeutic agents, which can potentially reduce treatment efficacy.

Cancer cells have a speedy rate of division; chemotherapy aims to target them while minimizing damage to normal cells. That leads to a lot of side effects like vomiting and diarrhea due to its impact on rapidly dividing healthy cells, such as those in the bone marrow, digestive tract, and hair follicles (hair loss).

In summary, chemotherapy plays a critical role in the comprehensive management of cancer, particularly when surgical options are limited or when addressing microscopic disease spread. Its success is influenced by tumor characteristics and requires careful planning to balance efficacy with quality-of-life considerations.

Radiotherapy Treatment

Radiotherapy is a foundation in cancer treatment, utilizing ionizing radiation to deliver a lethal dose to a defined tumor volume. The primary goal is to damage the DNA of cancer cells, particularly during mitosis, leading to cell death while minimizing harm to surrounding healthy tissues. This approach aims to eradicate the tumor and improve the patient's quality of life.

The effectiveness of radiotherapy depends on several factors, including the size, location, and appropriateness of the tumor for this treatment modality. Smaller, well-defined tumors are more amenable to precise radiation targeting, reducing the risk to adjacent normal tissues. Conversely, larger tumors or those located near critical structures may pose significant challenges, requiring advanced techniques such as stereotactic body radiotherapy (SBRT) to achieve optimal outcomes.

Advancements in radiotherapy have enhanced its precision and efficacy, allowing for higher doses to be delivered directly to the tumor while sparing healthy tissue. This precision reduces side effects and improves the overall effectiveness of the treatment.

In summary, radiotherapy plays a vital role in cancer management, particularly when tumors are appropriately sized and located for targeted treatment. Its ability to destroy cancer cells while preserving healthy tissue contributes significantly to tumor eradication and enhances the patient's quality of life.

Immunotherapy Treatment

Immunotherapy, also known as biological therapy, represents a revolutionary approach to cancer treatment by harnessing and enhancing the body's own immune system to recognize and destroy cancer cells. Unlike chemotherapy and radiation, which directly target and damage tumor tissue, immunotherapy works by awakening, stimulating, or restoring the immune system's natural ability to detect and eliminate malignant cells. Treatments include immune checkpoint inhibitors, monoclonal antibodies, cancer vaccines, and T-cell therapies such as CAR-T cell therapy. The effectiveness of immunotherapy can surpass that of traditional methods in certain cancers, such as melanoma, non-small cell lung cancer, kidney cancer, and some lymphomas, particularly when those tumors express high levels of neoantigens or PD-L1 proteins. However, its success depends significantly on the type of tumor, genetic markers, size, and location. For example, it may be less effective for tumors in immune-privileged sites, such as the brain, or for cancers with a low mutational burden. Nevertheless, for suitable patients, immunotherapy offers the potential for long-term remission and fewer side effects, making it a promising and often transformative option in modern oncology.

5.2 What are the side effects of conventional treatment

While conventional cancer treatment, such as surgery, radiotherapy, chemotherapy, and immunotherapy, can be highly effective in targeting and managing cancer, they often come with a range of short-term and long-term side effects due to their impact on both malignant and healthy cells.

Early side effects are common across treatments and include loss of appetite, nausea, vomiting, fatigue, neutropenia (a decrease in white blood cells, which increases the risk of infection), lymphedema (swelling due to lymphatic blockage), hair loss, and disturbances in sleep and mood, including depression. The severity and nature of these side effects often depend on the type and location of the cancer, as well as the treatment modality used.

Surgery, especially for internal organs, can result in postoperative infections, pain, scarring, and complications related to anesthesia. In some cases, microscopic cancer cells left behind may evade detection, leading to recurrence or metastasis.

Radiotherapy, though precisely targeted, can still affect surrounding healthy tissues, and prolonged exposure can lead to fibrosis, organ dysfunction, or even secondary cancers due to DNA damage in nearby non-cancerous cells. For example, radiation for breast cancer may incidentally affect lung or heart tissues, depending on the field of exposure.

Chemotherapy works systemically and targets rapidly dividing cells; however, in doing so, it also impacts healthy, fast-growing cells, such as those in the hair follicles, gastrointestinal tract, and bone marrow. This can lead to side effects such as mucositis, gastrointestinal distress, anemia, and increased susceptibility to infection. Furthermore, some chemotherapy-related side effects, such as cardiotoxicity or infertility, may manifest months or even years after treatment has ended.

Immunotherapy, while generally more selective, is not without risks. Its side effects are typically due to an overactivation of the immune system, potentially causing inflammation of organs (colitis, pneumonitis, or hepatitis), skin rashes, and thyroid or adrenal dysfunction. These immune-related adverse events, although less frequent, require careful monitoring and, in some cases, immunosuppressive treatment.

In summary, while conventional therapies are foundational in cancer management, understanding and proactively managing their side effects is essential for improving both quality of life and long-term outcomes in cancer care.

5.3 Tips to manage the side effects of conventional treatment

Undergoing conventional cancer treatments such as chemotherapy, radiation, and surgery can be physically and emotionally taxing. The side effects, ranging from nausea and vomiting to fatigue, hair loss, mood disorders, and digestive issues can impact daily living and overall well-being. However, with informed and practical strategies, many of these challenges can be effectively managed to support healing and resilience.

Nausea and vomiting can be alleviated by consuming small, frequent meals and drinking ginger-based teas or supplements. Avoiding greasy or overly sweet food helps, and some patients benefit from acupressure bands or prescribed antiemetic medications. To support blood count suppression, consume foods rich in iron (like leafy greens, lentils, and beets), vitamin B12, and folate. Juicing green vegetables, carrots, and apples can also deliver concentrated nutrients without burdening the digestive system.

Hair loss, though emotionally distressing, is often temporary. Cooling caps can reduce follicle damage during chemotherapy. Using mild shampoos and avoiding heat styling helps protect any remaining hair. For fatigue, rest is essential, but light physical activity, such as walking, yoga, or stretching, has been shown to improve energy levels and mood.

Mouth sores can be soothed with saltwater rinses and non-alcoholic mouthwashes. Avoid spicy or acidic foods during flare-ups. Loss of appetite is common, but juicing fruits and vegetables can provide vital calories and nutrients in a form that is easily digestible. Smoothies enriched with protein powder, flaxseeds, and nut butters can also help.

Diarrhea and constipation are side effects of both chemo and pain medications. For diarrhea, a low-fiber, BRAT diet (bananas, rice, applesauce, toast) is helpful, along with staying well-hydrated. For constipation, increase your dietary fiber intake, drink prune juice, and try warm lemon water. Rashes and dry skin respond well to natural moisturizers, such as aloe vera or calendula, and staying hydrated from within is crucial.

Pain, whether from surgery or tumor growth, should be addressed with both medical and non-medical interventions, like guided imagery, massage therapy, or warm compresses. Always consult your care team before taking over-the-counter pain relievers.

Mood disorders and depression are often overlooked. Psychological support through counseling, support groups, or therapy is essential. Meditation, journaling, and deep breathing exercises can also be powerful tools to regain emotional balance. Research suggests that depression may impact immune function, making emotional care as vital as physical treatment.

A holistic recovery approach should include detoxification and a clean, alkaline diet. Focus on whole, organic foods rich in antioxidants. Drinking alkaline water (pH 8-9.5), herbal teas, and fresh vegetable juices supports cellular health and toxin elimination. Ensure adequate sleep, as rest is critical for immune repair and mental clarity.

In summary, integrating traditional care with nutritional, emotional, and detox support can dramatically improve quality of life during cancer treatment. Empowerment comes from knowledge, and these practical steps can help patients feel more in control and supported on the path to healing.

Chapter 6:
Actionable Master Plan for beating cancer the natural way

Through the theories of cancer, we learned that several factors and conditions in our environment can cause us to have cancer; therefore, every person in their lifetime can develop precancerous cells in their body, but it is the decisions we make that affect our immune system and determine whether we get rid of the precancerous cells or develop a tumor. That means we must be careful about what we eat, drink, the environment we choose, and our emotional state. Our immune system is designed to identify and eliminate viruses, bacteria, etc., and when given the proper nutrition, our body can heal itself from cancer; the scientific community calls it spontaneous remission.

You must have a strong will to leave and be willing to change everything, with every bite you take in your life, you are building a new body. Ask your doctor if my cancer is fast-growing or slow-growing

6.1 Eliminating all the causes of cancer and committing to building a new body

A cancer diagnosis is a life-altering moment. While the shock is undeniable, what follows should be a period of deep reflection and honest self-inquiry. One of the most empowering steps a patient can take after diagnosis is to ask a vital question: How did this happen to me? This is not about blame, it's about clarity. Understanding and addressing the possible root causes of cancer in your life is not just wise; it may be essential to recovery.

Modern science increasingly supports the idea that cancer is a multifactorial chronic condition that results from a combination of internal vulnerabilities and external stressors, particularly long-term exposure to carcinogens or immune suppression conditions. Therefore, healing must start with the removal of the terrain that allowed the disease to thrive and the commitment to rebuild a new life.

This stage, radical self-inventory and elimination of root causes—is where transformation begins. It's the moment the light turns on. Every small step away from the causes of disease is a giant leap toward healing. By intentionally removing what no longer serves your health, you are giving your body the optimal conditions to repair, regenerate, and possibly recover more quickly and fully than you ever imagined.

6.2 Detoxifying the body: clear the path to recovery

Once you've taken a courageous inventory of your life, removed harmful inputs, and made a conscious decision to renew yourself, the next essential step is detoxification. We have a plethora of pathogens in our bloodstream, billions of them congested in our lymphatic system, pounds of purified waste stuck in our colon wall, causing these toxins to re-enter the bloodstream (autointoxication). We have billions of parasites living in our bodies, small pathogens like bacteria, viruses, and larger ones such as worms, invading our intestines, leaving toxic wastes in our bodies, and damaging our organs. Imagine a factory working 24 hours, overloaded but never stops for cleaning and maintenance. When your body is overloaded, it gets overwhelmed because the immune system cannot keep up with attacks. So, we want to reduce the toxic load and create an environment that is inhospitable to cancer. This starts with getting rid of these various pathogens in key areas like: blood, lymph nodes, colon, liver, and kidney.

What are some of the toxin burdens that must be removed?

Once you've taken a courageous inventory of your life, removed harmful inputs, and made a conscious decision to renew yourself, the next essential step is detoxification. Detox is not a trendy word or a crash diet; it's a biological reality, a continuous, intelligent function performed by your body every single second. But in today's toxic world, your body's natural detox systems are overwhelmed, and you must now give them strategic support to restore health.

What is the built-in Machinery working to detox you 24/7?

We need to think of our body as a high-performance engine that needs a clean oil filter to run efficiently. Your body needs its detox organs, especially the liver, kidneys, skin, lungs, and intestines, functioning optimally to remove waste.

The Liver is your body's primary detox engine. It breaks down harmful toxins, metabolic waste, pesticides, drugs, and chemicals, dumping many of them into the bile, which then moves into the intestines and out the "back door." The more you poop, the better your detox. Think of your liver as your internal oil filter,cleaning your blood and lymphatic system 24/7.

The Kidneys are your natural water purifiers. They filter your blood, removing waste and toxins that exit your body when you pee. Supporting your kidneys means drinking plenty of clean, mineral-rich water.

The Skin is your largest detox organ. Through sweating, you eliminate heavy metals, petrochemicals, and other fat-soluble toxins. Anti-perspirants and chemical-laden body care products block this vital channel, preventing toxins from exiting. Let your body sweat.

The Lungs are detox engines, too. Every time you breathe, your lungs convert and exhale toxins, especially carbon dioxide, a byproduct of cellular respiration. Clean, deep breathing helps you detoxify with every exhale.

The Colon must be cleared regularly. If bile and metabolic waste from the liver are not evacuated through the bowels, toxins are reabsorbed, a process called auto-intoxication. That's why regular, healthy bowel movements are essential.

Here's what you must begin removing:

- Processed and packed foods; refined sugar and high-fructose corn syrup; Trans-fats and hydrogenated oils; Red meat, processed meats (especially charred or nitrate-rich). All these are full of preservatives, additives, and synthetic chemicals that burden your liver and gut.
- Conventional produce laden with pesticides (opt for organic), herbicides, and Fungicides, heavily sprayed on non-organic crops, these are carcinogenic and endocrine-disrupting. For example, glyphosate (also known as Round-Up) is one of the worst offenders.
- Factory-Farmed Animal Products: These animals are fed pesticide-laced grains and injected with antibiotics and hormones. They accumulate toxins in their fat and organs, which you then consume.
- Tap water: often contains chlorine bleach (sodium hypochlorite) to kill bacteria and fluoride, which can damage neurological and immune health. These aren't needed for health; they're industrial chemicals.
- Mercury: A known carcinogen. Primary sources include vaccines, amalgam dental fillings (reservoir for chronic infection and systemic toxicity), and large fish like tuna. Tuna meat contains six times the safe mercury level. Mercury impairs immune function and mitochondrial health.
- Body Care Products: Lotions, creams, shampoos, and deodorants often contain parabens, phthalates, and petrochemicals, all absorbed through your skin and circulated through your bloodstream.

Master strategy to detoxify your body:

You don't fight toxins by doing nothing.

The first step is to start with a colonic (cleaning the colon wall from toxic materials stuck within, so it doesn't get reabsorbed in the bloodstream).

The second step is detoxifying the lymphatic system by killing off parasites and pathogens in the bloodstream and vital organs such as the liver, kidneys, and spleen. Here, the Beck protocol could be used or natural broad-spectrum binders that remove a variety of toxins from hepatic recirculation. Such binders are: ACTIVATED CHARCOAL, ZEOLITE, and SHILAJIT.

The third step is killing the parasites in the digestive tract.

Next, you dilute, flush, and mobilize them. Here's a practical and safe sequence to support deep detox:

1. **Hydration**: Start with a 3-day water fast if your health permits, or integrate alkaline water, herbal teas, and mineral broths to help your kidneys flush.
2. **Juicing**: Add **green juices** from cucumbers, celery, parsley, lemon, and ginger to alkalize and support the liver and gallbladder.
3. **Raw, Uncooked Foods**: Transition into a diet of raw vegetables and fruits. These are enzyme-rich and fiber-dense, helping to cleanse the gut and nourish your cells.
4. **Sweaty Exercise**: The lymphatic system, responsible for moving cellular waste, has no pump. You must move; rebounding, brisk walking, stretching, and deep breathing stimulate lymph flow and toxin removal.
5. **Chlorella**: This powerful green alga binds to heavy metals and toxins. Use a reputable brand, not from Japan, due to radiation exposure.

Chlorella contains chlorophyll, which helps cleanse the blood and support mitochondria.

By eliminating toxic inputs and supporting your body's natural detoxification, you change your internal environment—making it less favorable for cancer and more supportive of immune recovery. Healing is not just about adding medicine; it's about removing the burden. Once the body is unburdened, it can finally do what it was designed to do: heal itself

6.3 Detoxifying the mind: why stress is the invisible poison dampening healing

While detoxifying your body of toxins is essential in healing from cancer, detoxifying your mind is equally vital. Cancer is not just a physical disease; it can also be deeply rooted in emotional toxicity. Anger, bitterness, resentment, fear, worry, anxiety, insecurity, jealousy, envy, unforgiveness, and unresolved emotional trauma act like invisible poisons that weaken the body's ability to heal.

Stress isn't just "feeling tense"; it is a poison of the mind, a biological event triggered by the cocktail of emotions aforementioned, with powerful physiological consequences.

These emotions may feel normal in the chaos of modern life, but they signal danger to your brain and prevent your body from healing.

The Fight-or-Flight Hijack

When you experience these negative emotions, your brain activates the fight-or-flight response, a survival mechanism hardwired into your nervous system. Your body releases two key stress hormones:

- **Adrenaline**, which gives you temporary superhuman strength and sharp focus

- **Cortisol**, which signals your liver to release stored glycogen as **glucose**, pumping sugar into your bloodstream to fuel your muscles to either fight or flee

While acute stress is helpful in a real emergency (like escaping a wild animal), prolonged chronic stress turns this temporary state into a permanent mode of crisis.

In a chronic stress state, like living in constant fear, anxiety, or emotional pain, your body produces that excess cortisol and switches off or slows down your digestive system (nutrients aren't absorbed efficiently), your reproductive hormones are suppressed (fertility suffers), the reptilian instinctive part of your brain that allows you to think clearly, and that is why your thoughts get clogged up, you get stuck in a harmful loop and act like an animal, but sadly it switches your immune system too and you become vulnerable to opportunistic diseases and cancer.

Elevated cortisol also:

- Promotes inflammation, a well-known driver of cancer
- Increases abdominal fat, leading to insulin resistance
- Triggers weight gain and obesity, the second leading cancer risk factor after smoking

A study by Reiche et al (2004) that was published in *The Lancet Oncology* highlights that persistent activation of the HPA axis in depression likely impairs the immune response, contributing to cancer progression (30). Additionally, research from Stanford University School of Medicine found that women with breast cancer and depression exhibited altered immune cell activity, correlating with higher risks of cancer recurrence and mortality. These findings underscore the importance of addressing mental health in cancer care, as managing depression may enhance immune function and improve clinical outcomes.

Master Strategy to detoxify your mind

Detoxifying your mind starts with choosing emotional freedom:

- **Turn off the news cycle**: The 24/7 news cycle thrives on fear, drama, outrage, and repeated exposure to violent, depressing headlines that keep your nervous system on high alert.
- **Clean up your social feed and digital environment**: Constant exposure to negative posts, angry comments, or whining friends fuels inner stress
- **Unfollow unhappy, negative people** who complain or attack others and follow only those who inspire, uplift, and encourage healing
- **Identify and eliminate emotional vampires:** Some people consistently drain your energy through manipulation, drama, or constant crisis. These are *emotional vampires* you need to set boundaries and protect your space
- Practice forgiveness not for others, but for your healing
- Replace worry with faith and gratitude
- Turn guilt into self-compassion
- Replace bitterness with letting go
- Practice mindfulness
- Take nature walks
- Breathe deeply
- Build quiet moments into your day

This allows your body to shift from "fight or flight" into "rest and repair," the state where true healing happens.

You cannot heal in the same mental environment that made you sick. Detoxifying your body is not enough; your mind must be renewed, cleansed, and filled with peace, love, and hope. You must detoxify your thoughts, relationships, and emotional inputs. This is the foundation of long-term healing.

6.4 What healing supplement restores mitochondrial function and fuels cellular repair?

Once you've detoxified your body and begun to align your lifestyle for healing, the next powerful step in your journey is to restore your mitochondria, the energy factories of your cells. Mitochondria generate ATP, the energy currency your body needs to function, regenerate, and fight disease. In cancer, mitochondria are often damaged or dysfunctional, leading to disrupted energy metabolism and poor cellular communication.

Healing at the cellular level requires targeted nutrients that support mitochondrial health, improve immune function, reduce oxidative stress, and help your body reverse the damage done by chronic inflammation, toxins, and metabolic dysfunction.

Restoring healthy mitochondria not only strengthens every cell in your body but also starves cancer cells of the fermentation environment they thrive in.

Here are the supplements and natural compounds that can help rejuvenate your cells, boost immunity, and support cancer recovery, based on clinical experience, biochemical research, and anecdotal evidence from survivors.

1. Cesium Chloride and Potassium – Starving Cancer Cells of Energy

Cesium chloride is an alkaline mineral salt known for its controversial yet intriguing potential to raise intracellular pH, disrupting the acidic environment cancer cells depend on. When paired with potassium, this combination may help inhibit cancer cell metabolism by interfering with their energy production and nutrient absorption. Some alternative protocols have used cesium to help cancer cells absorb too much cesium, leading to cell death.

2. Vitality Formula – Cellular Energy and Repair (1 morning, one at lunch)

This supplement serves as your daily cellular vitality boost, combining coenzyme Q10, B-vitamins, adaptogens, and other mitochondrial nutrients that support:

- ATP production
- Cell membrane integrity
- DNA repair enzymes

These nutrients help the body generate clean energy while reducing oxidative damage.

3. Phyto-Defense – Anti-Cancer Plant Compounds (3 per day)

Packed with plant-derived antioxidants and phytochemicals, this supplement mimics the protective effect of a raw plant-based diet. Ingredients often include:

- Curcumin (from turmeric)
- Green tea extract
- Grape seed extract

These compounds reduce inflammation, block angiogenesis (tumor blood supply), and promote healthy cell signaling.

4. Vitamin E – Immune and Antioxidant Support (2 per day)

Vitamin E, particularly in its natural mixed tocopherol form, is essential for:

- Protecting cell membranes from oxidative stress
- Supporting immune modulation
- Improving circulation and tissue oxygenation

Its antioxidant power also protects healthy cells during cancer therapies.

5. Garlic – Natural Detoxifier and Cancer Inhibitor (9 capsules at night)

Garlic contains **allicin**, a powerful sulfur compound known for:

- Immune-boosting effects
- Anti-inflammatory action
- Inhibiting angiogenesis and tumor growth

Taken at night, garlic also helps detoxify heavy metals, support liver enzymes, and fight infections.

6. Zinc – Cellular Repair and Immune Shield (3 per day)

Zinc is crucial for:

- DNA synthesis
- Wound healing
- Enzyme activation
- Immune defense

It also plays a role in apoptosis (programmed cell death), a process that cancer cells often evade. Maintaining optimal zinc levels enhances immune surveillance of cancerous cells.

7. Aloe Vera Juice – Gut Healing and Anti-Tumor (6 ounces daily)

Aloe vera is more than just a soothing gel for skin. Internally, it:

- Soothes the GI tract
- Improves digestion and absorption
- Contains acemannan, a compound shown to stimulate macrophages and activate natural killer cells

Its gentle laxative effect also supports bowel detoxification, critical during cancer recovery.

8. Multi-Mineral Support – Replenishing the Foundations (4 per day; 2 AM, 2 PM)

Your body needs a full spectrum of minerals for every cellular function, including:

- Enzyme reactions
- Detoxification
- Mitochondrial enzyme cofactors

Key minerals like magnesium, selenium, chromium, and manganese are often depleted in people with cancer due to chronic stress and inflammation.

9. Salmon Oil – Anti-Inflammatory Omega-3s (2 per day)

Cold-water fish oils are rich in EPA and DHA, which:

- Lower inflammation
- Improve cell membrane fluidity
- Enhance brain function and mood

Omega-3s have been linked to reduced tumor growth and may make cancer cells more vulnerable to immune attack and apoptosis.

10. AHCC (Active Hexose Correlated Compound) – Immune System Commander

AHCC is a fermented extract from medicinal mushrooms, particularly *Lentinula edodes* (shiitake). It is a highly bioavailable alpha-glucan known for its ability to supercharge the immune system, a key defense mechanism against cancer cells.

Research shows AHCC:

- Boosts Natural Killer (NK) cell activity, the frontline soldiers that detect and destroy cancer cells
- Enhances dendritic cell response (immune messengers)
- Increases survival in cancer patients undergoing chemotherapy
- Modulates the balance of cytokines, reducing inflammation and supporting immune intelligence

Suggested dosage: 3g per day divided into two or three doses, best on an empty stomach

11. Vitamin C – Mitochondrial Ally and Antioxidant Guardian

Vitamin C (ascorbic acid) is a powerful antioxidant with dual roles in cancer therapy:

- At low to moderate doses, it protects healthy cells from oxidative damage caused by free radicals and treatment side effects.
- At high doses (intravenous Vitamin C), it behaves like a pro-oxidant in cancer cells, generating hydrogen peroxide inside tumors that selectively kills cancer cells without harming normal tissue.

Key benefits of Vitamin C in cancer recovery:

- Stimulates collagen synthesis, crucial for tissue repair
- Enhances iron absorption and detoxification pathways
- Regenerates other antioxidants like glutathione and Vitamin E
- Supports adrenal function and reduces fatigue
- Improves quality of life during chemotherapy or radiation

Suggested dosage:

- **Oral**: 2,000–5,000 mg daily in divided doses with meals

- **IV (clinically supervised)**: 25,000 to 75,000 mg per session, depending on individual protocol

Caution: Avoid high-dose Vitamin C if you have G6PD deficiency, kidney disease, or oxalate sensitivity. Always consult a healthcare provider before starting IV protocols.

Bonus Tip: Stack Smart for Maximum Impact

Some of these compounds work synergistically. For example:

- **Vitamin C + AHCC** = Enhanced immune intelligence and protection from oxidative stress
- **Zinc + Vitamin E + Omega-3s** = Anti-inflammatory cellular repair matrix
- **Chlorella + Garlic + Aloe Vera** = Detox support and gut healing

Conclusion

Consistency and commitment to a lifestyle are key to detoxifying and strengthening the body, the mind, uplifting the spirit, and healing from cancer. Each supplement listed above contributes uniquely to your body's battle. They don't work in isolation, but in harmony—like instruments in an orchestra—amplifying your innate capacity to heal when you nourish, protect, and energize your cells.

If you forgot everything we discussed above, here is the simplified action plan drawn from this chapter:

1. Nourish with Healing Foods

- Drink a fresh vegetable juice daily (ginger root, turmeric root, lemon, carrots, celery, cucumber, red and green cabbage, and a touch of apple for flavor).

- Eat only organic, non-GMO whole foods. Avoid processed, packaged, canned, frozen, and restaurant foods.
- Prefer cooking methods such as boiling, slow cooking, grilling, or broiling.
- Eliminate refined carbohydrates and sugars. Instead, if needed, choose wild rice, organic beans, or lentils.
- Avoid seed oils and fast food entirely.

2. Reset the Metabolism

- Practice intermittent fasting (e.g., dinner at 6:30 p.m. and breakfast at 10:30 a.m.).
- Start the day with lemon water made from freshly squeezed lemon in purified water.
- Take ½ teaspoon of organic baking soda each morning to support alkalinity.

3. Natural Healing Supports

- Drink 6 ounces of Aloe vera per day
- Drink soursop tea regularly.
- Consume 5 apricot seeds, three times daily.
- Follow an antioxidant and nutrient program to boost immunity and aid detoxification.
- Consider antiparasitic support (e.g., ivermectin), as some cancers may be linked to hidden infections.

4. Remove Hidden Toxins

- Detoxify your living environment by replacing toxic personal care and household products (shampoos, conditioners, detergents, soaps, shaving gels, deodorants, toothpaste, skin creams) with safe, natural alternatives.

5. Supplements

- Take 3 Phyto-defense per day
- Take 2 Vitamin E per day
- Take 9 Garlic cloves at night
- Take 3 Zinc per day
- Take 2 Salmon oil pills a day

6. Important tips when you have Cancer

- Sunshine (Vitamin D for immune function. We get through sun exposure)
- Water (Hydration to keep body fluid clean and alkaline)
- Air (oxygen therapy, breathe and clear your mind)
- Rest (Recover Energy Strength Time)
- Exercise (move your body and lymph)
- Laughter (It releases endorphin through the brain, do some silly and laugh)
- Food (get all nutrients for bigger impact, let food be your medicine)

Detox (through your skin, lungs, liver, colon, and kidneys)

Chapter 7:
Survivor Stories and the Science Behind Their Success

7.1 Jocelyn healing stage IV Colon Cancer through nutrition-based therapy

When Jocelyn, a 49-year-old mother of three from California, was diagnosed with stage IV colon cancer, the Doctors told her that the tumor had spread to her liver and lymph nodes, and her chances of long-term survival were slim. Jocelyn underwent surgery to remove part of the colon, but when chemotherapy was offered as the next step, she hesitated. She had seen what aggressive chemotherapy had done to her sister, ravaging her body while buying her only a few more months of life. Jocelyn felt she needed a different path. In her words: *"I wanted to heal, not just fight. I wanted to give my body the tools it needed to recover instead of destroying what little strength I had left."*

Jocelyn opted for a nutrition-based therapy that emphasized plant-based, organic foods, freshly pressed juices, detoxification, and natural supplements. She committed to the following:

Diet & Juicing: She consumed nearly 20 pounds of organic fruits and vegetables daily, mostly through freshly pressed juices every hour. These juices delivered concentrated enzymes, antioxidants, and nutrients that nourished her body and supported detoxification.

Detoxification Protocols: She practiced coffee enemas multiple times a day. Though controversial, Jocelyn believed they helped her liver flush toxins, reducing nausea and restoring energy.

Supplements: She integrated natural compounds like pancreatic enzymes, minerals, and vitamins to strengthen her immune system and support cellular repair.

Lifestyle Shift: Jocelyn eliminated all processed foods, sugar, and animal protein. She dedicated herself to rest, gentle movement, prayer, and stress reduction.

The first few months were grueling. She lost weight, her family doubted her choices, and she experienced detox crises that felt like setbacks. But slowly, her energy returned. After one year of unwavering discipline, follow-up scans revealed that her tumors had shrunk significantly to what her oncologist described as "unexpected" and "highly unusual" remission.

Jocelyn is now cancer-free and continues to follow a modified version of her healing protocol, maintaining her plant-based lifestyle, daily juicing, and seasonal detox routines. She has become an outspoken advocate for integrative cancer care, often telling audiences:

"I am living proof that when you give your body the right conditions, it knows how to heal itself."

Here is the Science behind Jocelyn's Healing Story

1. Nutrient Density & Cellular Repair

Jocelyn's consumption of enormous amounts of fresh, organic fruits and vegetables through juicing provided her body with concentrated phytonutrients, antioxidants, vitamins, and minerals in a highly bioavailable form.

- These nutrients play key roles in DNA repair, mitochondrial function, and reducing oxidative stress, which are critical in cancer recovery.

- For example, compounds like sulforaphane (from cruciferous vegetables) and quercetin (from apples and onions) have been shown to suppress cancer cell growth and activate detox enzymes.

2. Mitochondrial Support

Cancer is increasingly understood as a metabolic disease at its core, where damaged mitochondria push cells toward abnormal fermentation (the Warburg effect).

- A plant-based, low-toxin diet rich in raw enzymes helps restore mitochondrial function by reducing the metabolic load (less sugar, fewer toxins) and supplying cofactors like magnesium, B vitamins, and coenzyme Q10 that mitochondria need.

3. Detoxification & Liver Support

The liver is the body's main detoxification hub. Coffee enemas, though controversial, are believed to stimulate bile flow and glutathione production, enhancing the body's ability to neutralize free radicals and clear toxins.

- By reducing toxic burden, the immune system can redirect energy toward healing rather than constant firefighting.

4. Immune System Reboot

A clean diet and detox protocols may lower chronic inflammation (measured through markers like CRP and cytokines).

- By lowering inflammation and providing immune-supportive compounds (like vitamin C, beta-glucans, and selenium), the body's natural defenses can more effectively target abnormal cancer cells.

5. Fasting-Mimicking State

Even though Jocelyn wasn't fasting in the traditional sense, consuming high amounts of raw plant-based foods creates a low-insulin, low-IGF-1 environment conditions under which cancer cells struggle to thrive, but normal cells adapt and survive.

Research on fasting and caloric restriction shows these metabolic states can sensitize tumors to die off while protecting healthy tissue.

6. Mind-Body Healing

Chronic stress fuels cancer through cortisol spikes, immune suppression, and systemic inflammation. Jocelyn's shift toward meditation, prayer, and rest likely rebalanced her nervous system, supporting overall recovery.

7.2 David Turning the Tide against Advanced Metastatic Prostate Cancer

David was 58 when he heard the words no man wants to hear: *"It's advanced, metastatic prostate cancer."* The cancer had spread to his bones and lymph nodes, and the prognosis was grim. His oncologist recommended immediate hormone therapy and chemotherapy, but David, a retired engineer, wanted more than just extending life—he wanted to restore health.

Instead of surrendering to despair, David decided to become an active participant in his healing journey. He studied tirelessly, discovering emerging research on how nutrition and metabolism influence cancer growth. What struck him most was the idea that cancer feeds on sugar and thrives in an inflamed, nutrient-poor environment.

David overhauled his lifestyle overnight. He switched to a strict ketogenic diet, eliminating all refined sugars, grains, and processed foods. His meals centered around organic vegetables, healthy fats like olive oil, avocado, and coconut oil, and moderate portions of grass-fed protein. By drastically lowering carbohydrates, David aimed to starve his cancer of glucose while fueling his healthy cells with ketones.

He also began daily juicing, flooding his body with nutrients from green vegetables, ginger, turmeric, and herbs. While he avoided fruit juices due to sugar, he crafted blends that delivered concentrated antioxidants and anti-inflammatory compounds to support his immune system.

In addition, David practiced intermittent fasting, eating only within a 6-hour window each day. Twice a month, under medical supervision, he embarked on 72-hour water fasts to push his body into deep autophagy—the natural "clean-up" process that removes damaged cells and stresses cancer metabolism.

The first months were difficult. David lost weight rapidly, and at times he doubted himself. But gradually, his energy returned stronger than before. He noticed the chronic pain in his hips easing. His blood markers, including PSA levels, began dropping. Follow-up scans showed something even more astonishing: the cancer in his bones had stabilized, and some lesions had even regressed.

His oncologist, initially skeptical, was stunned. After two years of strict adherence to his nutritional protocol, David's scans showed no active evidence of disease progression. He was living not just longer, but better walking daily, gardening, and playing with his grandchildren without pain.

David calls his recovery *"a second chance."* He often tells other men facing prostate cancer:

"I didn't cure my cancer with a magic bullet. I changed the environment in which it lived. I stopped feeding it and started nourishing myself. My body did the rest."

Here is the Science behind David's Healing

David's recovery can be better understood through the lens of the metabolic theory of cancer, or a disease of disordered cellular energy metabolism. David created a metabolically hostile environment while supporting his body's innate repair and immune metabolism. Here's how his strategies likely worked together:

1. Ketogenic Diet – Starving Cancer Cells of Sugar

- **Normal cells** can adapt to using ketones (from fat) as fuel.
- **Cancer cells**, however, rely heavily on glucose fermentation (the **Warburg effect**) because of damaged mitochondria.
- By drastically lowering carbohydrate intake, David reduced glucose **and insulin availability**, making it harder for cancer cells to thrive while strengthening healthy cells.

Ketones themselves may even act as signaling molecules that reduce inflammation and oxidative stress.

2. Intermittent Fasting & Extended Water Fasts – Triggering Autophagy

- Fasting lowers insulin and IGF-1 (growth signals that drive tumor growth).
- Extended water fasts trigger autophagy, a cellular recycling process that clears out damaged components and may eliminate pre-cancerous or weak cells.

- Fasting also stresses cancer cells, which cannot adapt well to low-glucose, low-growth-factor environments, while normal cells enter a protective "survival mode."

3. Juicing – Flooding the Body with Phytochemicals

- David's green juices provided concentrated polyphenols, flavonoids, and antioxidants from plants like kale, ginger, and turmeric.
- Compounds such as sulforaphane (broccoli), curcumin (turmeric), and quercetin (greens) have been shown in lab studies to:
- Suppress tumor-promoting inflammation
- Induce apoptosis (programmed cancer cell death)
- Support detoxification pathways in the liver
- Juicing allowed him to consume far more micronutrients than by eating vegetables alone.

4. Reduced Inflammation & Strengthened Immunity

- Chronic inflammation is a key driver of prostate cancer progression.
- The ketogenic, plant-rich diet helped reduce systemic inflammation, lowering cytokines and oxidative stress.

Fasting periods improved immune surveillance, giving his body's natural killer (NK) cells and T-cells a better chance to identify and destroy cancer cells.

5. Metabolic Reprogramming of the Tumor Environment

- By removing sugar spikes, lowering insulin, and sustaining ketone levels, David changed the tumor microenvironment.

Cancer thrives in an acidic, glucose-rich environment. Instead, his body shifted toward a low-glucose, ketone-fueled, oxygen-rich state, a setting that is far less favorable for cancer cell growth and spread.

7.3 Sarah's Story: Defying the Odds with Metastatic Breast Cancer

In January 2022, Sarah, a 49-year-old mother of two, sat in her oncologist's office staring at a report that felt like a death sentence. Her cancer tumor marker was 776, a shocking number. The scans confirmed her breast cancer had metastasized to her lungs. Her doctor gave her a prognosis no one wants to hear: *"You may only have a month to live."*

But Sarah refused to accept that this was the end of her story. Instead of collapsing into despair, she made a bold decision to take radical ownership of her healing journey. Rather than relying solely on conventional medicine, she chose a holistic path, drawing strength from nature, nutrition, faith, and family.

Her Healing Action Plan

Sarah knew she couldn't wait. She transformed her lifestyle overnight:

Nutrition reset: She went completely vegan—cutting out all meat, sugar, refined carbs, and processed food. Every bite was intentional fuel for her healing.

Juicing therapy: She flooded her body with fresh, organic juices, especially green juices packed with broccoli, kale, and spinach.

Garlic power: Each night, she ate nine raw garlic cloves, believing in their natural anti-cancer and immune-boosting properties.

Aloe vera & clean food: She drank aloe vera juice daily and committed to only non-GMO, organic foods.

Lifestyle healing: She prioritized sleep, deep rest, exercise, sunshine, fresh air, and pure water.

Spiritual renewal: Sarah dedicated time each day to prayer, gratitude, and connection **with her family**, nourishing her soul as much as her body.

The Results

Her results stunned everyone.

- After just **3 months**, her tumor marker **dropped from 776 to 225**.
- At the **6-month mark**, it fell again to **40**.
- She was now **just a step away from the "normal" range of under 38 U/ml**.

Her oncologist, who once doubted she would live beyond a month, now had to acknowledge something extraordinary had happened. Sarah's body healed itself not miraculously, but systematically, through the natural tools she had given it.

The Science behind Sarah's Recovery

1. Plant-Based Vegan Nutrition

- **No meat, no sugar, no refined carbs** → These are the foods that fuel inflammation and insulin spikes. High insulin and glucose availability directly promote cancer growth (the *Warburg Effect*). By cutting them out, Sarah deprived her cancer cells of their preferred fuel.
- **Plant-rich diet** → Flooded her body with phytonutrients, antioxidants, vitamins, and minerals. Compounds in cruciferous vegetables like **broccoli** (sulforaphane) and **kale** activate detox pathways and can trigger apoptosis (programmed cancer cell death).
- **Fiber-rich foods** → Improved gut health, which is increasingly tied to immune system regulation and cancer defense.
- **Juicing Therapy**
- Fresh vegetables and green juices deliver a **concentrated dose of micronutrients** that bypass digestion and are rapidly absorbed.

- For example, **carrot juice** (rich in beta-carotene) and **beet juice** (high in betalains and nitrates) have documented anti-cancer and blood-oxygenating effects.
- Juicing also supports **detoxification** by providing enzymes that aid the liver in neutralizing carcinogens

3. Garlic (9 cloves nightly)

- Garlic contains **allicin** and sulfur compounds, which are strongly linked to anti-cancer properties.
- Studies suggest garlic can:
- Inhibit carcinogen activation
- Induce apoptosis in cancer cells
- Reduce angiogenesis (formation of new blood vessels feeding tumors)
- The "massive dose" Sarah took was essentially using food as medicine.

4. Aloe Vera Juice

- Contains **acemannan**, a polysaccharide shown to **stimulate the immune system**, increasing activity of macrophages and natural killer (NK) cells.
- Aloe also has **anti-inflammatory** and **gut-healing** effects, improving nutrient absorption and overall resilience.

5. Lifestyle Healing (Sleep, Exercise, Sunshine, Fresh Air, Clean Water)

- **Sleep**: During deep sleep, the body releases melatonin, a hormone with **anti-cancer properties** (it suppresses tumor growth and scavenges free radicals).
- **Exercise**: Increases circulation, oxygen delivery, and immune surveillance (making it harder for tumors to thrive in low-oxygen environments).

- **Sunshine**: Boosts **vitamin D**, critical for immune regulation and cancer prevention. Low vitamin D is strongly correlated with worse outcomes in breast cancer.
- **Fresh air & clean water**: Reduce toxic burden and improve oxygenation. Since cancer thrives in low-oxygen (hypoxic) environments, a better oxygen supply may slow tumor growth.

6. Spirituality, Family, and Emotional Healing

- Chronic stress and fear elevate cortisol and weaken the immune system. Sarah's **spiritual practices, prayer, and family support** activated what researchers call the **"relaxation response"**, lowering stress hormones and improving immune function.

Psychoneuroimmunology studies show that hope, connection, and spiritual belief can boost NK-cell activity, directly improving cancer defense.

7. Tumor Marker Drop Explained

- The fall from **776 → 225 → 40** in six months suggests:
- Reduction in systemic inflammation.
- Slowing of tumor metabolism due to glucose deprivation and nutrient environment changes.
- Enhanced immune recognition and clearance of cancer cells.
- Her results line up with the concept of metabolic reprogramming: she changed the internal environment of her body from cancer-friendly to cancer-hostile.

Key Takeaway

Sarah's recovery was not "miraculous" in the supernatural sense—it was biological and systematic. By addressing:

- Metabolism (starving cancer of sugar/fuel),

- Detoxification (through juices, garlic, aloe),
- Immunity (via nutrition + stress reduction),
- Environment (oxygen, vitamin D, rest), she created conditions where her body could fight back and heal itself.

7.4. Anecdotal story of Alina defying Appendix Cancer

Alina, a 52-year-old teacher, was experiencing symptoms like pelvic cramping, bloating, skin changes, and irregular menstrual cycles. These symptoms led her to a CT scan that revealed a mass on her appendix. Diagnosed with stage 4 appendix cancer, Alina underwent surgery to remove her appendix. However, by this point, the cancer has spread to other organs, including her liver, her diaphragm, uterus, bladder, and ovaries. Alina continued the battle with additional surgeries and many rounds of chemotherapy. Unfortunately, two years into her struggle, her oncologist told her to get her affairs in order as the cancer was way too advanced and she only had six weeks left. However, Alina wanted to live to see her daughter graduate from high school. Instead of surrendering to hospice, Alina took massive action and embarked on a new path of self-empowerment, focusing on repairing the powerhouses of her cells (mitochondria) through nutrition and targeted adjuncts.

Alina's Nutritional Protocol

Alina designed her meals to provide her body with compounds known to reduce oxidative stress, support DNA repair, and promote apoptosis (programmed cell death).

- **Green Juices and Liquid chlorophyll**: every day she drank at least one liter of green juices made with spinach, kale, lettuce, artichoke, collard greens, and drank liquid chlorophyll before bed
- **Cruciferous vegetables**: she ate a lot of Broccoli, cabbage, cauliflower, and Brussels sprouts to modulate a detox pathway, protect her DNA, and support cellular resilience.

- **Colorful antioxidants**: Blueberries, pomegranates, turmeric, and green tea were included daily to counteract free radical damage.
- **Healthy fats**: Extra virgin olive oil, avocados, and omega-3-rich foods like flaxseed helped her strengthen cell membranes.
- **Intermittent fasting**: Alina practiced intermittent fasting to boost her mitochondrial efficiency.
- **Protein balance**: She relied on plant proteins, nuts, and no red meat, focusing instead on amino acids from cleaner sources.

Integrating Repurposed Medicines

Alongside nutrition, Alina integrated Ivermectin & Fenbendazole compounds for their anti-cancer properties, following the below dosage:

- **Ivermectin**: 1 mg/kg/day
- **Fenbendazole**: 444 mg/day, taken six days a week

Emerging studies suggest that these two medicines interfere with microtubule formation and cancer cells, and by combining them with her nutrition plan, Alina gave her body an extra shield.

Results

Six months after following the above strict regimen, Alina's scans and bloodwork started to show improvements, her disease stabilized, her energy returned, and she regained control over her daily life.

A year later, Alina's scans and bloodwork showed no evidence of cancer. Alina believed what cured her cancer was the synergy: *nature's pharmacy in cruciferous vegetables and antioxidants to restore her cells, plus the ivermectin–fenbendazole combination to target malignant pathways.*

The Science behind Alina's Recovery

Alina's story reflects an integrative approach, nutrition to strengthen her body at the cellular level, combined with repurposed medicines that have drawn interest in cancer research.

1. Nutrition and Mitochondrial Support

- **Liquid chlorophyll**: Used for detoxification, research at the Oregon State University Linus Pauling Institute shows that chlorophyll reduces biomarkers of aflatoxins, binds to carcinogens in the gut, and blocks their absorption.
- **Green Juicing**: Daily consumption of fresh green juice provides the cells with high concentrations of vitamins A, C, K, minerals, and phytochemicals to support immune function
- **Cruciferous vegetables (broccoli, cabbage, cauliflower, Brussels sprouts):** These contain *sulforaphane* and *indole-3-carbinol*, compounds that can activate detoxification enzymes, reduce oxidative stress, and influence epigenetic expression linked to DNA repair.
- **Antioxidants (berries, green tea, and turmeric):** Help neutralize free radicals, lowering the burden of oxidative DNA damage that fuels cancer progression.
- **Mitochondrial health:** Intermittent fasting and polyphenol-rich foods promote *autophagy* (the clearance of damaged cellular components) and improve mitochondrial efficiency — supporting the body's natural defense systems.

2. Repurposed Medicines – Ivermectin & Fenbendazole

- **Ivermectin:** Traditionally an antiparasitic, some preclinical research suggests it may inhibit cancer cell proliferation by blocking *P-glycoprotein* (a drug resistance pump), altering energy metabolism, and disrupting key survival pathways in tumor cells.
- **Fenbendazole:** A veterinary anthelmintic shown in laboratory studies to destabilize microtubules in cancer cells, much like certain chemotherapy drugs, leading to apoptosis (programmed cell death).

3. The Synergy of Both Approaches

By restoring her cellular health with nutrition while introducing repurposed agents that may disrupt malignant signaling, Alina essentially built a **two-pronged defense system**:

Strengthen the healthy cells so they can resist damage.

Weaken cancer cells by disrupting their survival mechanisms.

7.5 Karla's Story: Choosing Life Again after recurring Metastatic Breast Cancer

In 2003, Karla received the news every woman dreads: she was diagnosed with breast cancer. At the time, she followed the conventional medical path: surgery, chemotherapy, and radiation. The treatment was grueling, but it worked. Karla went into remission, and for the next eleven years, she lived cancer-free. Life slowly returned to normal until one day, it didn't.

In 2014, Karla's cancer came back. This time, it had spread. Her diagnosis was metastatic breast cancer, and doctors told her it was incurable. The prognosis was grim, but Karla refused to accept that this was the end of her story. Instead, she made a life-changing decision: to take massive action and address every aspect of her life, body, mind, and spirit.

Karla embarked on a holistic healing journey. She transformed her nutrition and lifestyle, began deep emotional healing, and opened herself to spiritual growth. She learned to listen to her body and to treat it with compassion rather than fear. Through forgiveness, she released old wounds and emotional burdens that had weighed her down for years. She often referred to forgiveness as her greatest medicine.

Along the way, Karla embraced new daily practices that strengthened her inner peace. Meditation, prayer, and gratitude became her foundation. She learned to "break up with busy," creating space for rest, joy, and presence. She also surrounded herself with love and support, both from her community and from a deepening connection to divine guidance. Bit by bit, she rebuilt her life around healing rather than fighting.

These profound changes created what Karla calls a "body no longer hospitable to cancer." Against all odds, her health has steadily improved, and since 2016, she has shown no evidence of disease.

Today, Karla has turned her journey into purpose. She is a cancer coach, co-founder of Health Navigator, a virtual cancer wellness community, and co-director of the Radical Remission Project, helping others discover their own pathways to healing and hope. Her life is a testament to the power of belief, love, and the human spirit's capacity to heal.

Karla's story reminds us that while we may not always choose our challenges, we can always choose our response, and in that choice lies the potential for transformation.

The Science behind Karla's Healing

Karla's recovery from metastatic breast cancer is remarkable, and while such outcomes are uncommon, they are not without precedent. In recent years, a growing body of evidence has begun to illuminate the biological mechanisms that may help explain how comprehensive lifestyle and mind-body interventions can influence cancer progression and overall health.

1. The Mind–Body Connection

Research in psychoneuroimmunology has shown that emotional states and chronic stress can directly affect immune function. Prolonged stress elevates cortisol and inflammatory cytokines, which can suppress the body's natural ability to detect and destroy malignant cells. Practices such as meditation, prayer, and emotional release have been shown to reduce stress hormone levels, lower inflammation, and enhance immune function. (Sources: Ader & Cohen, 1993; Black & Slavich, 2016; Antoni et al., 2006)

2. Nutrition and Cellular Environment

Diet plays a powerful role in shaping the body's internal terrain. Studies suggest that anti-inflammatory, plant-forward diets rich in antioxidants and phytonutrients can decrease oxidative stress, modulate gene expression, and improve metabolic health, creating conditions less favorable for cancer growth. By focusing on nutrition as medicine, Karla supported her body's innate repair systems. (Sources: Ornish et al., 2005; Campbell & Campbell, 2006; Katz & Meller, 2014)

3. The Role of Emotional Healing and Forgiveness

Emotional trauma and unresolved resentment have been linked in research to physiological stress responses and immune suppression. Acts of forgiveness and emotional release can shift the nervous system from chronic "fight-or-flight" mode toward balance, promoting healing on a systemic level. (Sources: Toussaint et al., 2015; Worthington & Scherer, 2004)

4. Spiritual Connection and Purpose

Spirituality and a sense of purpose have been repeatedly correlated with improved quality of life and even survival in cancer patients. Feelings of connection — to community, to meaning, to the divine — can buffer stress, foster resilience, and influence behaviors that promote healing. (Sources: Puchalski et al., 2014; Koenig, 2012)

5. Lifestyle Medicine and Epigenetics

Perhaps most compelling is the emerging evidence that lifestyle changes can influence gene expression, turning on genes that protect health and turning off those that promote disease. Research by Dr. Dean Ornish and colleagues has demonstrated that diet, exercise, stress reduction, and social support can lead to beneficial changes in gene activity within months. (Sources: Ornish et al., 2008; Blackburn & Epel, 2012)

Karla's story for defeating a metastatic recurring cancer highlights the potential of the holistic, a whole-person approach, one that integrates body, mind, and spirit to complement medical care. Science continues to uncover how factors like mindset, nutrition, emotional healing, and connection can create a biological environment more conducive to recovery and long-term wellness.

Karla's experience serves as a living example of what can happen when evidence-based medicine and the healing power of human consciousness meet.

7.6. Murrays' Story – From Terminal Kidney Cancer to Thriving

At the age of forty-three, Murray was having blood in the urine and severe back pain. After several scans, he received the devastating diagnosis of stage IV renal cell carcinoma, an aggressive form of kidney cancer. Surgeons removed his kidney, but soon after, the cancer had metastasized to his lungs, liver, and abdomen. When doctors informed him that there were no further medical options for him after more rounds of chemo, Murray faced what most would consider the end of the road.

But Murray refused to accept this prognosis. Instead, he made a conscious decision to take charge of his own healing. What followed was a radical transformation of body, mind, and spirit. He adopted a whole-food, plant-based diet, incorporated daily juicing, and prioritized rest, meditation, and deep spiritual work. He also supported his recovery with herbal supplements, including five tablets of IP6 800 mg & 5 tablets of Inositol 220 mg, taken in the morning and at night. He surrounded himself with an environment of hope, peace, and gratitude.

Over time, Murray's strength returned, his energy grew, and follow-up scans revealed something extraordinary: his cancer was gone. Against all odds, Murray became completely **cancer-free**.

Today, Murray and his wife, Mags, have turned their remarkable journey into a mission. Together, they run a holistic healing retreat in England, where they teach others the same principles that restored Murray's health and transformed their lives. His story stands as a powerful testament to the resilience of the human spirit and the body's innate capacity to heal when nourished with faith, love, and intention.

The science behind Murray's story

Murray's recovery illustrates the profound biological changes that occur when the body's internal environment is shifted toward healing. Modern research supports that a **whole-food, plant-based diet** can reduce systemic inflammation, lower oxidative stress, and enhance immune function, all key factors in slowing or even reversing disease progression.

Daily juicing and nutrient-rich foods supply powerful antioxidants and phytochemicals that help neutralize free radicals and support cellular repair. Meanwhile, **meditation, rest, and stress reduction** are known to lower cortisol levels and promote parasympathetic nervous system activity, allowing the body to focus energy on regeneration rather than defense.

As far as the supplements go, here are the main biological mechanisms by which the combination of IP6 + inositol has been shown to act in pre-clinical cancer models:

1. **Cell-cycle arrest and inhibition of proliferation.** IP6 has been shown to increase expression of cyclin-dependent kinase inhibitors and reduce the activity of CDKs/cyclin complexes, leading to G1 phase arrest in cancer cells.
2. By reducing proliferative signaling, the tumor cells are slowed in their division.
3. **Induction of apoptosis (programmed cell death) and autophagy.** Several studies show that IP6 induces apoptotic pathways: for example, in prostate carcinoma cells, IP6 treatment led to caspase-3 activation, PARP cleavage, down-regulation of survival signals, and mitochondrial pathway involvement.
4. In one colon cancer model, IP6 inhibited the PI3K/Akt/mTOR pathway and triggered autophagy-mediated cell death
5. **Inhibition of key signaling pathways in cancer survival and angiogenesis.** IP6 suppresses the PI3K/Akt pathway, leading to reduced phosphorylation of downstream targets. It also reduces angiogenic markers in tumor xenografts, thereby potentially limiting tumor blood supply.
6. **Modulation of extracellular matrix, cell adhesion, migration, and metastasis.** In one breast cancer model, IP6 reduced the expression of specific integrin receptors. It inhibited focal adhesion kinase signaling, thereby reducing cancer cell adhesion to the extracellular matrix and limiting migration/invasion.
7. In colon cancer metastasis models, IP6 plus inositol reduced liver metastases and altered the expression of matrix metalloproteinases (MMPs), fibronectin, laminin, etc.
8. **Antioxidant, immune-modulating, and differentiation effects. Some review articles suggest that IP6 may enhance antioxidant enzyme activity, reduce lipid peroxidation,** and enhance immune surveillance (e.g., increased NK cell activity) in animal/experimental models. WAOCP Journal+2PubMed+2

9. IP6 + inositol has been shown in some models to induce differentiation of malignant cells (i.e., revert them toward more normal behavior) rather than merely killing them. PubMed+1

7.7. Louis' Story – From Death Sentence to New Life

Louis, a friend from South Africa, became one of the greatest inspirations, mentors, and nutrition coaches in my cancer journey. At just 26 years old, Louis was diagnosed with leukemia. For five long years, he and his medical team tried everything conventional medicine had to offer, every drug, every medication, and every treatment available. Eventually, his doctors told him the words no one wants to hear: "We cannot help you anymore." Sent home with nothing but a death sentence, Louis could have given up. But then, a friend introduced him to a different way of thinking, that the body itself is the healer when given the right conditions.

Louis made a radical decision to change his lifestyle. He removed toxins and poisons from his environment, cleansed and detoxified his body, and rebuilt his health from the inside out. He began juicing daily with powerful blends of ginger root, turmeric root, lemon, carrots, celery, cucumber, red and green cabbage, with a touch of apple for flavor. He committed to eating only fresh, organic, non-GMO whole foods — nothing boxed, canned, frozen, or from restaurants. He practiced intermittent fasting, drank lemon water, and prepared simple boiled or slow-cooked meals. He eliminated processed carbohydrates, refined sugars, seed oils, and toxic household products, replacing them with natural alternatives. His regimen also included apricot seeds, soursop tea, baking soda, supplements, antiparasitic support, and a focused antioxidant program to boost immunity.

By creating an environment that allowed his body to heal, Louis transformed his life. What was once a hopeless diagnosis turned into a testimony of strength, discipline, and faith. Today, Louis is cancer-free, living proof that resilience, determination, and holistic healing can open doors when conventional medicine closes them. His journey has made him not only a survivor but also a source of wisdom, guidance, and hope for others walking the same path.

Louis' secret protocol for Healing from Cancer

1. **Daily Vegetable Juice** – Freshly pressed juice every day, made with ginger root, turmeric root, lemon, carrots, celery, cucumber, red cabbage, green cabbage, and a small amount of apple for flavor.
2. **Eat Only Organic, Non-GMO Foods** – No boxed, canned, frozen, or processed foods. Cook everything from scratch: no restaurant or fast food.
3. **Intermittent Fasting** – Dinner at 6:30 p.m. and breakfast at 10:30 a.m. the next day.
4. **Lemon Water** – Fresh lemon squeezed into purified water daily.
5. **Whole Food Meals** – Simple boiled stews, crockpot cooking, grilled or broiled meals using whole, organic ingredients.
6. **Eliminate Processed Carbohydrates** – No rice, pasta, bread, flour, sugar, or fruit juices. If craving carbs, only eat wild rice, organic beans, or lentils.
7. **Detox the Body and Home**–Remove all toxic personal care and household products, including shampoos, conditioners, laundry detergents, skin creams, dishwashing soaps, shaving gels, deodorants, and toothpaste.
8. Replace with natural, toxin-free alternatives.
9. **Baking Soda** – Half a teaspoon of organic baking soda every morning.
10. **Soursop Tea** – Drink regularly as part of the healing plan.
11. **Apricot Seeds** – Eat five apricot seeds, 3 times per day.
12. **Parasite Cleansing** – Take ivermectin to address potential parasite-related cancer triggers.
13. **Antioxidant Nutrient Program** – Support the immune system, detox the body, and fight cancer naturally with targeted supplements.
14. **No Seed Oils** – Eliminate refined or industrial seed oils.

The Science behind Louis' Recovery

Louis' transformation was not simply a matter of chance — many of the steps he took are supported by scientific understanding of how lifestyle, nutrition, and detoxification influence the body's healing potential.

1. **Nutrient-Dense Juicing** – Fresh vegetable juices provided his body with concentrated vitamins, minerals, antioxidants, and phytochemicals such as sulforaphane (from cabbage and cruciferous vegetables), curcumin (from turmeric), and gingerol (from ginger). These compounds are known to reduce inflammation, neutralize free radicals, and support the liver's natural detoxification pathways.
2. **Eliminating Processed Foods & Toxins** – By removing processed foods, refined sugar, seed oils, and chemical additives, Louis reduced the burden of toxins and inflammatory compounds that can weaken the immune system. Studies consistently show that diets high in whole, organic, plant-based foods lower cancer risk and improve cellular repair.
3. **Intermittent Fasting & Metabolic Health** – His fasting routine gave his digestive system regular rest, reduced insulin spikes, and may have promoted **autophagy** — the body's natural process of cleaning out damaged cells, including potentially precancerous or cancerous ones.
4. **Detoxification of Body and Home** – Our skin and lungs absorb many of the chemicals from household and personal care products. By eliminating these exposures, Louis reduced his toxic load, freeing his immune system to focus on repair and recovery.
5. **Herbal and Natural Support** – Soursop leaves, apricot kernels (containing amygdalin), and antioxidant supplements are all used in various natural healing traditions. While evidence varies, many plant-based compounds demonstrate antioxidant, anti-inflammatory, or antiparasitic effects that may support the body's resilience.
6. **Immune System Strengthening** – Ultimately, Louis' plan worked to create an internal environment that supported his immune system. By

fueling his body with whole foods, eliminating toxins, and maintaining a healthy metabolic rhythm, his natural defenses were strengthened to do the work they were designed to do: fight disease and restore balance.

7. Louis' recovery illustrates a powerful scientific truth: when the body is nourished, cleansed, and supported, its innate healing mechanisms can be activated in profound ways.

Disclaimer:

Louis and other patients' stories and healing plans are personal testimonies of their journeys with cancer. Such action plans reflect individual choices and experiences, and are shared here for inspiration and educational purposes. They are not a substitute for medical advice, diagnosis, or treatment. Anyone facing a cancer diagnosis or health condition should consult qualified healthcare professionals before making changes to their diet, supplements, or lifestyle.

1. **The Ketogenic Diet**: One of the most promising dietary approaches for supporting mitochondrial health is the ketogenic diet. By drastically reducing carbohydrate intake and increasing healthy fats, the body shifts to using ketones for fuel. Ketones are a cleaner energy source that produces fewer free radicals during metabolism, reducing oxidative stress on the mitochondria.

2. *Practical Step*: Start by eliminating processed sugars and grains. Gradually increase the intake of avocados, coconut oil, fatty fish, and nuts to promote a state of ketosis.

3. **Intermittent Fasting (IF)**: Another powerful tool is intermittent fasting, which helps initiate autophagy—the body's natural process for clearing out damaged cells and regenerating healthier ones. This practice allows for more efficient mitochondrial recycling and repair.

4. *Practical Step*: Begin with a simple 16:8 fasting schedule (16 hours of fasting followed by an 8-hour eating window). This can boost metabolic flexibility and mitochondrial function over time.

5. **Targeted Supplementation**: Nutritional supplements can provide the building blocks necessary for mitochondrial repair. Maria's regimen included Coenzyme Q10 (CoQ10) for energy production, alpha-lipoic acid (ALA) as an antioxidant, and resveratrol for its anti-inflammatory properties.
6. *Practical Step*: Consult with a healthcare provider to determine appropriate dosages. Supplements should be high-quality and taken consistently for the best results.

Turning point in all patients' anecdotes

After a few months of implementing these strategies, patients described waking up in the morning feeling an unusual surge of energy, a stark contrast to the fatigue that had become their norm. Later on, laboratory tests revealed improved markers of oxidative stress and mitochondrial function.

Practical Tips

- **Stay Consistent**: Nutritional changes require time to show results. Stick to a regimen for at least 3-6 months for noticeable improvements.
- **Monitor Progress**: Work with your healthcare team to track biomarkers like oxidative stress levels and mitochondrial efficiency.
- **Listen to Your Body**: Adjust dietary and fasting practices based on how you feel and respond.

The Science-Backed Hope

Emerging studies from institutions such as the Department of Energy's SLAC, National Accelerator Laboratory, and Stanford University have shown that repairing mitochondria can improve the body's natural defense mechanisms. The combination of the ketogenic diet, intermittent fasting, and targeted supplementation provides a robust, practical framework to address metabolic dysfunction.

Our survivors' journeys have illustrated that by prioritizing mitochondrial health, we empower our bodies with the tools needed to fight not just cancer, but a host of metabolic diseases. The path to healing lies in the commitment to understanding and nurturing our cellular engines, one step, one meal, and one day at a time.

Metabolic Pathways and Microbial Influence: Rethinking Cancer through Nutrition and Parasitic Parallels

The Effect of Dietary Proteins on Enzyme Activity

Research (74–75) demonstrates that higher protein consumption increases the activity of mixed-function oxidase enzymes, primarily located in the liver. These enzymes play a central role in metabolizing various substances, including potential carcinogens. Conversely, a low-protein diet reduces enzyme activity, which can limit the binding of carcinogens to DNA, thereby decreasing carcinogen activation, tumor growth, and interference with detoxification processes. This highlights the critical balance between dietary protein intake and the body's enzymatic defense mechanisms against cancer development.

Implications of the Microbiota in Cancer Drug Metabolism

The absorption and bioavailability of orally administered drugs are regulated by both host and bacterial enzymes within the intestines (42). However, certain medicines and xenobiotics can, in turn, alter the gut microbiota's composition and gene expression, indirectly modifying how drugs are metabolized.

Notably, antiparasitic drugs such as Ivermectin and Fenbendazole have attracted attention for their off-label exploration in cancer research. These compounds bind to glutamate-gated chloride channels, leading to parasite death, and disrupt microtubule formation, an essential process in cell division.

If cancer cells share fundamental metabolic similarities with parasites, therapeutic strategies traditionally used against infections may hold potential in oncology. By targeting shared metabolic pathways and survival mechanisms, researchers could uncover innovative treatment modalities. This intersection between oncology and parasitology invites a re-evaluation of cancer's underlying biological processes, fostering a deeper understanding of its complexity and revealing new avenues for intervention.

Chapter 8:
Role and Importance of Integrative Approaches (Holistic Cancer Treatment)

Integrative oncology is a new and humane science that combines modern medicine with the wisdom of nutrition, mind-body practices, energetic balance, and personalized care. While traditional oncology focuses on removing the mass or tumor caused by cancer, the integrative approach focuses on the terrain or means of repairing the patient's inner environment to eradicate cancer growth. Instead of asking "How can we kill these cells?" we begin to ask:

- Why did these cells lose their regulatory signals?
- What in the metabolic, immune, or energetic landscape allowed this breakdown?
- How can we restore internal coherence so that healthy cells thrive and malignant cells fade?

In this model, conventional treatments such as surgery, radiation, immunotherapy, and chemotherapy are no longer the only tools in the healing orchestra. Instead, they are supported, balanced, and amplified by nutrition, detoxification, stress reduction, and energetic therapies.

For a better understanding of how the integrative approach works, some more profound questions must be investigated, such as: what is cell oscillation, vibration, or communication in the mitochondria, and what causes the body to lose its ability to recognize and repair itself?

To understand how cancer starts, we must picture the roles of the different organelles in our cells. For lack of a better illustration, if we draw a parallel at the macro level to organs in the human body, we have organs such as the liver, kidneys, lungs, etc.

Just as the liver in the human body maintains blood glucose while the kidneys maintain fluid balance, organelles in the cell allow the cell to function correctly. In our cells, we have two prominent organelles: the nucleus and the mitochondria. The mitochondria make the energy to enable the body to produce ATP. Mitochondria have their own genetic material that operates independently of nuclear DNA.

There is a rhythm to life far deeper than the heartbeat; in fact, every cell hums with a quiet vibration, a symphony of electric potentials, ionic waves, and molecular resonance. When that rhythm is intense and harmonious, life expresses health, vitality, and balance. When it becomes discordant, the melody fades into disease.

1. The Vibrational Nature of Life

Every living system oscillates. From the heartbeat and circadian rhythm to the flow of ions across membranes, oscillation is the language of life. Inside the cell, mitochondria generate bioelectric potentials, creating faint electromagnetic fields that pulse in time with metabolic activity. These fields are not random noise they're information.

A healthy mitochondrion oscillates at a balanced "frequency" of energy production. This is not a musical tone, but a biophysical rhythm of voltage and redox state, a pattern that reflects coherent ATP synthesis, efficient electron flow, and balanced reactive oxygen species (ROS). When mitochondria are synchronized, they form networks of resonance. Their inner membranes pulse in harmony, exchanging energy, calcium, and redox signals. It's like an orchestra: when every instrument is tuned, the music flows effortlessly. But when one instrument falls out of tune, when a mitochondrion "buzzes wrong," the dissonance can spread.

2. When the Buzz Turns Toxic

Every mitochondrion both senses and emits subtle signals — electrochemical, photonic, and even acoustic at the nanoscale. When energy flow is disrupted, whether by nutrient deficiency, oxidative stress, or viral interference, a mitochondrion begins to misfire.

Instead of a steady rhythm of electron transport and ATP production, it begins to leak electrons, overproduce ROS, and lose its membrane potential. The result is a distorted vibration, a buzz that's both a symptom and a signal. And because mitochondria communicate, that signal spreads.

Through fusion and fission dynamics, through ROS diffusion, through calcium waves, a single dysfunctional mitochondrion can entrain its neighbors into chaos just as one detuned violin can throw an entire quartet off balance. In this way, disease propagates not only through mutation but also through communication.

Cells with chaotic mitochondrial oscillations lose redox control, shift into anaerobic metabolism (the Warburg effect), and begin to proliferate uncontrollably. The loss of bioenergetic coherence becomes the seed of malignancy.

3. Mitochondria: The Cellular Internet

Mitochondria don't work in isolation. They are nodes in a living web that constantly fuse, divide, and exchange information. Through nanotubular connections, mitochondria can move between cells, carrying not just energy but also signaling molecules, mtDNA, and metabolic states.

In health, this intercellular sharing supports repair and adaptation. In a disease, it can spread dysfunction. A population of healthy mitochondria vibrates coherently, a distributed intelligence balancing oxidation and reduction, charge and discharge, rest and action. But when dysfunction spreads, it's like a viral meme, an alarming frequency that synchronizes more and more cells into chaos. Seen this way, cancer is not a solitary event, but a breakdown of the community, a loss of coherence among the cell's energy nodes.

4. Out-of-the-Box Therapeutic Thinking

If cancer is fundamentally a loss of coherence, then restoring coherence may be a key to healing. This means going beyond the traditional "kill the tumor" approach and instead restoring the vibrational harmony of the cellular ecosystem. Some emerging and speculative approaches include:

1. **Bioenergetic tuning:** Interventions that restore mitochondrial membrane potential and ATP balance — from metabolic therapies (fasting, ketogenic diets, and NAD^+ boosters).

2. **Redox rebalancing:** Using mitochondrial-targeted antioxidants (like MitoQ or SS-31) not to suppress ROS entirely, but to restore their rhythmic signaling pattern.

3. **Mitochondrial biogenesis and fusion support:** Activating pathways like PGC-1α and SIRT1 through exercise, fasting, or specific nutraceuticals (resveratrol, CoQ10) to encourage mitochondrial network reconnection — reestablishing communication.

4. **Electromagnetic coherence therapy (emerging):** Research into how low-intensity electromagnetic fields, sound, or light frequencies might help realign cellular oscillations — a frontier still in its infancy, but conceptually consistent with restoring mitochondrial rhythm.

5. **Viral detoxification and immune recalibration:** Addressing chronic viral latency (HSV, HPV, and EBV) that keeps mitochondrial signaling

disturbed, through immunomodulation, antiviral nutrients, and mitochondrial resilience enhancement.

These strategies do not "attack" cancer directly. They **tune the system** supporting the body's own intelligence to restore order from chaos.

Nutrition as Medicine

Food is the most consistent biochemical message we send to our bodies. Every meal can either inflame or calm, feed cancer or starve it, disrupt mitochondrial function or restore it. We must understand that every breath of energy serves as an acceptor, allowing the cell to function, just as an oxygen spark ignites combustion. As cancer cells are addicted to Glucose and Glutamine, for example, the best way to deal with cancer is to pull the plug on these two fermentation fuels. Key integrative nutritional strategies include:

a. Metabolic Nutrition

- Ketogenic and low-glycemic diets limit glucose, the preferred fuel of many cancer cells, and can push cells toward oxidative metabolism.
- Fasting-mimicking diets and intermittent fasting enhance autophagy (cellular cleanup), reduce insulin and IGF-1 signaling, and may make tumors more sensitive to therapy.

b. Phytonutrients and Antioxidants

- Compounds like curcumin, EGCG (green tea), resveratrol, and sulforaphane support detoxification, modulate inflammation, and restore redox balance.
- However, antioxidant use must be personalized — excessive supplementation during specific therapies can blunt treatment efficacy.

c. The Mitochondrial Diet

- Focus on whole, living foods: colorful plants, omega-3 fats, organic proteins, and fermented foods that nourish mitochondrial function and gut microbiota.
- Avoid refined sugars, processed oils, and toxins that disturb cellular communication.

Food is not merely fuel; it is information. Each nutrient whispers instructions to your genes and mitochondria: "repair," "adapt," "grow," or "rest."

Anticancer activities of Cannabinoids and how they regulate mitochondria

Cannabinoids have been studied for their effects on oxidative phosphorylation, a crucial step in mitochondrial cellular respiration. Cannabinoids may regulate mitochondrial function by modulating the electron transport chain, thereby supporting oxidative phosphorylation.

Reduction of Reactive Oxygen Species (ROS): Cannabinoids can help reduce the production of reactive oxygen species, byproducts of cellular metabolism that can cause oxidative stress and cell damage.

Modulation of Energy Homeostasis: Cannabinoids also interact with the endocannabinoid system, which regulates energy balance and metabolism at the cellular level. Cannabinoids may regulate mitochondrial function by influencing the activity of the electron transport chain, thereby supporting oxidative phosphorylation.

Detoxification and Cellular Cleansing

The modern environment overwhelms us with toxins heavy metals, plastics, pesticides, and pollutants. These compounds accumulate in fatty tissues, interfere with mitochondrial enzymes, and increase oxidative stress.

Integrative cancer programs often include:

- Gentle detoxification: infrared saunas, lymphatic massage, Epsom salt baths, and hydration.
- Liver support: nutrients like N-acetylcysteine, alpha-lipoic acid, milk thistle, and glutathione.
- Colon and lymphatic cleansing to improve elimination and immune function.

Detoxification is not a single event; it's a rhythm, a cellular breathing. When you restore that rhythm, your body's natural repair processes reactivate.

The Mind–Body Connection

Cancer is not only biological; it is emotional and energetic. Chronic stress, trauma, and unresolved emotions activate the hypothalamic-pituitary-adrenal (HPA) axis, flood the system with cortisol, and suppress immune surveillance.

Research now confirms that mind-body medicine directly influences tumor biology:

- Meditation and mindfulness lower stress hormones and inflammation.
- Yoga, qigong, and tai chi improve circulation, lymphatic flow, and energetic coherence.
- Breathwork increases cellular oxygenation and calms the nervous system.
- Psychotherapy, especially trauma-informed or somatic-based therapies, helps release the stored tension that can perpetuate disease.

Healing the mind is not an optional extra, it is a biological necessity

The Energy Medicine Perspective

Beyond biochemistry lies bioenergetics, the field of energy flow that governs all physiological processes. Every cell, every mitochondrion, vibrates with an electromagnetic rhythm. When stress, toxins, or infection disrupt these rhythms, the body's natural order begins to break down.

Integrative energy-based modalities include:

- Acupuncture and acupressure, balancing meridian energy and modulating immune response.
- Low-level laser and photo-biomodulation therapy, restoring mitochondrial energy and reducing inflammation.
- Pulsed electromagnetic field (PEMF) therapy improves cellular communication and membrane potential.
- Sound therapy and frequency-based medicine, still experimental, but aiming to re-harmonize disordered vibrational patterns.

These methods are not meant to replace conventional treatment, but to **reconnect the body's information network**, allowing it to regain coherence.

The Role of the Microbiome and Immunity

Nearly 70% of the immune system resides in the gut. When the microbiome is diverse and balanced, it trains immune cells to distinguish friend from foe, healthy from malignant. When it is imbalanced (dysbiosis), inflammation rises, and immune tolerance breaks down.

Integrative protocols support immune recovery through:

- Probiotics and prebiotics
- Fermented foods like kefir, kimchi, and miso

- Fiber-rich, plant-based diversity
- Stress reduction and adequate sleep, both of which profoundly affect the microbiome

The goal is to create an **internal ecology** that is unfriendly to cancer but nurturing to regeneration.

Targeting Mitochondrial and Metabolic Health

At the deepest level, cancer reflects a loss of mitochondrial coherence, the breakdown of the cell's energy control center. Integrative oncology works to retune this energy system through:

- Nutrient cofactors: magnesium, CoQ10, carnitine, B-vitamins, and NAD^+ boosters.
- Oxygenation therapies: ozone (in some protocols), hyperbaric oxygen, and deep breathing.
- Redox balance restoration through both nutrition and lifestyle.
- Exercise and movement, which stimulate mitochondrial biogenesis and repair.

Movement, sunlight, grounding, and even laughter are signals to the mitochondria that life is safe, that energy can flow freely again.

Spiritual and Existential Healing

Many survivors speak of a profound inner transformation in that cancer became not just a biological event, but a call to awaken. Integrative medicine honors this spiritual dimension.

Healing often involves:

- Forgiveness of others, of oneself.
- Reconnection to meaning and purpose.
- Gratitude practices, prayer, and meditation.
- Deep listening to the body's wisdom.

When the spirit realigns with life's purpose, biology often follows.

Closing thoughts on the integrative approach for curing cancer

The fight against cancer demands an integrative understanding of human metabolism connecting nutrition, energy balance, hormonal regulation, and cellular bioenergetics.

In healthy physiology, the body has remarkable metabolic flexibility: it can use glucose as its primary fuel, but in conditions of low carbohydrate intake or fasting, the liver produces ketone bodies. B-hydroxybutyrate and acetoacetate as efficient alternative energy molecules. These ketones not only support normal tissues such as the brain and muscles but also modulate oxidative stress, inflammation, and cellular signaling pathways. Unlike glucose, ketones produce less reactive oxygen species, potentially reducing DNA damage and mutational burden.

Cancer cells, due to mitochondrial dysfunction and reliance on glycolysis (the "Warburg effect"), are often less capable of utilizing ketones for energy. This opens a therapeutic window: promoting metabolic states in which normal cells thrive on ketones, while cancer cells struggle to adapt, may enhance treatment outcomes or reduce recurrence risk. This is not a replacement for conventional therapy but a metabolic complement, part of a broader integrative strategy.

Cure in integrative oncology does not mean merely removing a mass; it means restoring the terrain for life to thrive. When the mitochondria hum again in their perfect rhythm, when energy flows freely, and the inner environment is restored, the body remembers its song. And in that remembrance, victory becomes not only possible but inevitable. Victory over cancer is not just the absence of disease. It is the presence of harmony where every cell, every mitochondrion, every thought vibrates with the frequency of balance and vitality.

Chapter 9:
How To Stay In Control and Prevent Recurrence

Victory over cancer is not only about treatment, but it is the beginning of a new way of living. The body you now inhabit has been through fire and has come out transformed. Your immune system has learned, your metabolism has changed, and your spirit has grown resilient. However, we need to be mindful that cancer stem cells are very slick in evading traditional therapies such as chemotherapy and radiation because they target the tumor and do not necessarily prevent relapse. After successful treatment, the mission does not stop here; we must continue monitoring our bodies to avoid any possibility of recurrence by destroying cancer stem cells at the roots. This means creating and nurturing an internal environment or terrain that is hostile to cancer stem cells, forcing them to self-destruct rather than enter a dormant or more resistant state. The new terrain rewires cancer cells to "activate cell death," ensuring the disease cannot take root there again.

9.1 Long-term health monitoring

After remission, your greatest ally is consistent monitoring. Regular checkups, screening, blood panels, imaging when indicated, and biomarker testing are not reminders of fear; they are affirmations of strength. They say, "I am paying attention." They allow your care team to spot small changes before they become significant, and they keep you connected to your recovery story. Healing doesn't end when the scans turn clear; it evolves into lifelong vigilance, a partnership between self-awareness and science.

9.2 Turning your bloodstream into a hostile ground for cancer stem cells

The chemo and radiation did their job by killing more than 95% of the cancer. The patient entered remission, and the cancer appeared to have gone away, but it may come back because it still has the mutation that drove the disease in the first place. Modern research has revealed that what we call "cancer" is often sustained by these small, stubborn populations of cancer stem cells (CSCs), the seeds of recurrence. The few stragglers, stem cells, or leftovers that still harbor cancer will start growing again: one becomes two, two becomes four, and so on. Usually, these cells are now resistant to the type of chemo or radiation you used because they have adapted.

Our bodies shed about sixty billion blood and gut cells, which new ones replace through a natural process called apoptosis. After treatment, the goal is to create a blood environment where cancer stem cells cannot thrive.

The secret is metabolic harmony: keeping inflammation low, energy balanced, and oxidative stress under intelligent control. Several natural and pharmaceutical compounds have shown promise in studies aimed at influencing this microenvironment.

We do not know of any cancer of any kind that can survive without Glucose and Glutamine; by keeping this in mind, it becomes clear how to manage and prevent cancer recurrence. Cancer patients can use nutrition, supplements, and non-toxic medication to block sources that fuel cancer. Treatment to inhibit the use of glucose and prevent glycolysis includes prescription medication such as:

Low-Dose Tadalafil (Cialis): As a repurposed drug, low-dose Tadalafil, which is usually used to treat erectile dysfunction, has shown remarkable potential in cancer treatment. Tadalafil works by inhibiting the enzyme PDE5, increasing nitric oxide levels, and improving blood flow, thereby decreasing inflammation, enhancing immune cell infiltration, and improving the body's ability to attack CSCs.

Statins and Statin-like compounds: Statins influence lipid pathways, known for lowering cholesterol, and can impact CSCs by blocking the mevalonate pathway, which is crucial for CSC growth. By doing so, statins weaken CSCs and prevent them from proliferating.

Metformin supports insulin sensitivity and energy regulation.

The nutrients listed below, such as high-dose vitamin C and flavonoids abundant in fruits, teas, and plants, are being studied for their potential to disrupt cancer stem cell survival.

Flavonoids: found in colorful fruits, green tea, cocoa, and citrus peel, have antioxidant and signaling properties that may help balance cell growth and immune tone.

Pectin: a soluble fiber abundant in apples and citrus, has been studied for its ability to bind certain galectins, molecules linked to cell adhesion and metastasis. Pectin, just like the ascorbic acid below, lowers cholesterol and disrupts CSC growth while combating inflammation and oxidative stress, supporting the body's fight against cancer.

Vitamin C (ascorbic acid), especially at higher dietary intake levels, supports immune vigilance and mitochondrial function.

Citrus Bergamot: the fragrant, aromatic fruit with a bitter taste originating from southern Italy, no bigger than an orange, has drawn attention for its unique flavonoid profile, and can support cholesterol balance, metabolic flexibility, and antioxidant defense. This food possesses several statin-like properties due to its high levels of polyphenols and flavonoids. Bergamot is so special because, in addition to flavonoids, it contains pectin and ascorbic acid, making it uniquely effective against CSC.

The point here is not to self-prescribe, but to understand which molecule or meal you can put into your system to shift your internal chemistry toward health.

Grounding, Movement, and Connection: You are an electrical being living on an electrical planet. Practices like grounding or earthing, spending time barefoot on natural ground, and allowing the body to exchange subtle electrical charge with the Earth are being studied for their potential effects on inflammation and stress recovery. Grounding decreases inflammation by lowering cortisol levels, a stress hormone that promotes inflammation. Grounding improves sleep and enhances mood, boosts immune function, reduces chronic pain, enhances blood circulation, which helps deliver oxygen and nutrients to cells more efficiently, and promotes tissue repair and healing.

Whether through grounding, yoga, walking, or mindful breathing, what matters is that you reconnect your body to the natural, circadian, and emotional rhythms. A body in rhythm resists chaos.

9.3 Rebuilding the terrain: metabolic health as prevention

Cancer risk and recurrence are closely tied to metabolic diseases, obesity, insulin resistance, and chronic inflammation. The same conditions that fuel diabetes can silently encourage cancer stem cells to awaken. Your defense is metabolic clarity:

- Favor whole, unprocessed foods rich in fiber and phytonutrients.
- Maintain stable blood sugar through consistent meal timing and balanced macronutrients.

- Keep body fat within a healthy range — not out of vanity, but out of vigilance.
- Support restorative sleep and active circulation, because oxygen and movement starve stagnation.

9.4 Tips to block sources that fuel cancer

Food will become more than nourishment. After remission, you want to choose only meals that will keep inflammation low. Fill your plate with deeply colored vegetables and fruits: the blues, the greens, and the reds that can flood your bloodstream with antioxidants and polyphenols.

The danger of animal products: Switch to a plant-based diet that is rich in whole foods low in processed or refined sugar, as meta-analysis research shows that animal products (beef, pork, lamb), processed food, and sugar drive chronic inflammation linked to cancer, diabetes, and heart diseases (Larsson & Osini, 2014).

Cooking Meat at High Temperature: Heterocyclic amines (HCAs) and polycyclic aromatic hydrocarbons (PAHs) are chemicals formed when muscle meat, including beef, pork, fish, or poultry, is cooked using high-temperature methods, such as pan frying or grilling directly over an open flame (Cross & Sinha, 2004).

Do not consume processed foods: What characterizes these types of foods is the injection of Trans fat, artificial additives, refined sugar, high levels of sodium, and several unhealthy chemicals to preserve their longevity on the shelf, which is proven to promote chronic inflammation (BMJ, 2019).

Do not consume refined sugars: The American Journal of Clinical Nutrition found that consuming refined sugars, especially fructose and sucrose, triggers the production of fatty acids in the liver, leading to increased inflammation markers and compounds, including CRP

(American Journal of Clinical Nutrition, 2014). Trade refined sugar for fibers and healthy fats from olives, nuts, and seeds, which steady insulin and calm metabolic fires.

<u>Consume Flaxseed:</u> The flaxseed consumption appeared to lower the cancer-cell proliferation rates, while at the same time increasing their rate of cancer-cell clearance (Demark, 2001).

<u>The benefits of broccoli-family (cruciferous) vegetables:</u> Certain compounds in broccoli have been proven to have a suppressive effect on cancer metastasis. In a 2010 study, scientists laid down a layer of human lung cancer cells in a petri dish and cleared a swath down the middle. Within twenty-four hours, the cancer cells had crept back together, and within thirty hours, the gap had closed completely. But when the scientists dripped some cruciferous vegetable compounds onto the cancer cells, the cancer cells ' creep was stunted. Cruciferous vegetables, in general, like broccoli, kale, and Brussels sprouts, are nature's detox engineers.

<u>Carcinogen-blocking effect of Turmeric:</u> Since 1987, the National Cancer Institute has tested more than a thousand different compounds for "chemopreventive" (cancer-preventing) activity. Only a few dozen have made it to clinical trials, but among the most promising is curcumin, the bright-yellow pigment in turmeric. The anticancer effects of curcumin extend beyond its ability to prevent DNA mutations potentially. It also appears to help regulate programmed cell death. Your cells are preprogrammed to die naturally to make way for fresh cells through a process known as apoptosis (from the Greek ptosis, "falling," and apo, "away from"). In a sense, your body is rebuilding itself every few months (16), with the building materials you provide through your diet. Some cells, however, overstay their welcome—namely, cancer cells. By somehow disabling their own suicide mechanism, they don't die when they're supposed to. Because they continue to thrive and divide, cancer cells can eventually form tumors and potentially spread throughout the

body. Curcumin can also kill cancer cells directly by activating "execution enzymes" called caspases, which destroy them from within by cleaving their proteins (18). In a last-ditch attempt to save the lives of fifteen patients with advanced colorectal cancer who didn't respond to any of the standard chemotherapy agents or radiation, oncologists started them on a turmeric extract. In the two to four months of treatment, it appeared to help stall the disease in one-third of the patients, five out of fifteen (18).

Chapter 10:
Call To Action and Resources For Further Reading

As we come to the end of this book, I want to leave you with a truth, and that is: healing is possible. No matter how dark the diagnosis, no matter how heavy the burden, within each of us lies an extraordinary power to heal, to rebuild, and to live again. Cancer may have entered your life, but it does not define your future. The stories you've read, stories like Murray's, remind us that the body's capacity to recover is far greater than we have been led to believe. But healing is not passive. It is a conscious decision, made day after day, to choose life.

Your healing journey begins with what you feed your body and your mind. The foods you eat, the thoughts you think, and the peace you allow yourself to feel these are not small things. They are medicine.

10.1 Taking Control of Your Health

The moment you decide to take control of your health is the moment cancer loses its most significant advantage, fear. Cancer thrives in silence, in waiting, in surrender. But when you step forward, informed and intentional, you become the architect of your own recovery. Taking control isn't about defiance; it's about awakening. It's the realization that your body is not your enemy but your most powerful ally, waiting for your partnership and attention.

True healing begins when you shift from being a passive patient to an active participant. That means learning your numbers, understanding your treatments, asking questions, and building a relationship with your care team that is based on knowledge, not intimidation. It means seeing every test, every choice, and every day of wellness not as a chore but as a declaration of ownership over your life.

Taking control also extends beyond the clinic. It lives in your daily habits in the food you choose, the sleep you protect, the movement you practice, and the peace you cultivate. You may not have chosen this fight, but you can choose how you fight it. When you nourish your body with real foods, strengthen it with movement, and calm your mind through rest and gratitude, you send a clear message to your cells: *We are living, not merely surviving.*

There will be moments when fatigue whispers, and doubt lingers, but control is not perfection; it is persistence. It's showing up for yourself one meal, one breath, one checkup at a time. Each small action is a brick in the fortress you're building a life that cancer cannot easily breach.

Taking control of your health is not about fear of recurrence; it's about the joy of stewardship. You are the guardian of your own vitality, and every choice you make from the water you drink to the thoughts you entertain writes the story of your continued victory.

10.2 Trusted Resources and Support Networks

Trusted Resources and Support Networks

When you're navigating your life beyond treatment, making informed choices is your strongest ally. This means turning to resources you can trust, connecting with communities who understand, and building a network of support that honors your unique path. Below are curated

organizations, websites, and networks that offer credible information, emotional comfort, and practical guidance, especially relevant if you're exploring nutritional or integrative strategies alongside standard care.

1. National and Trusted Information Hubs

National Cancer Institute (NCI): The U.S. government's leading cancer-research institute. Use it for authoritative overviews of treatments.

The National Center for Complementary and Integrative Health (NCCIH) is a credible resource for complementary approaches (nutritional strategies, supplements, lifestyle) and for what the research says (and doesn't) about them.

American Cancer Society (ACS) offers robust patient programs, educational materials, online communities, and helplines.

2. Support Groups and Community Networks

CancerCare.org provides free counseling, support groups (online, phone, in-person) for survivors and caregivers, with a focus on emotional and practical support.

Cancersupportcommunity.org offers virtual programs, peer networks, and education focused on wellness after cancer.

3. Nutrition and Integrative-Health Guides

Mahealth.org focuses on diet, exercise, and recovery.

Dana-farber.org The Academy of Nutrition & Dietetics' oncology-nutrition website "Eat Right to Fight Cancer."

4. Some resources to explore before trying nutritional or alternative approaches

Visit cancerresearchuk.org to understand popular diets or supplements (ketogenic, alkaline, etc.) through the lens of rigorous evidence.

Always check with your oncologist or integrative medicine specialist before introducing new compounds or supplements to ensure they do not interact negatively with your treatment.

Get information only from reliable websites ending in ".gov", ".edu", and well-known ".org".

For a cancer patient, resources are lifelines that remind you that you are not alone, that your curiosity and questions are valid, and that science, networks, and community support your journey toward sustained health. As you walk this path, draw on these trusted sources to guide you with clarity and confidence and let them become part of your personal victory over cancer.

10.3 Final Words of Encouragement

If there is one message I would like you to take from Victory over Cancer, it is this: never surrender your hope. Healing begins the moment you believe it is possible. Every breath is a chance to start again. Every meal, every walk, every moment of gratitude is a step toward a new life.

You are not a victim of disease; you are a partner in your healing. You are not powerless; you are the most crucial participant in your recovery. And you are not alone; there is a growing global community of survivors, healers, and seekers walking this path with you.

The Next Chapter Is Yours

This is not the end of your story. It is the beginning of your victory. The body can heal, the spirit can rise, and life can bloom again in ways you never imagined.

So continue being courageous, stay disciplined, and spend each moment with love.

Feed your body with living foods.

Feed your mind with hope and truth.

Feed your spirit with peace and purpose.

And remember always: You are stronger than cancer. You are life itself, resilient, radiant, and victorious.

Selected References

1. Cross AJ, Sinha R. Meat-related mutagens/carcinogens in the etiology of colorectal cancer. *Environmental and Molecular Mutagenesis* 2004; 44(1):44–55.
2. Red Meat and Processed Meat consumption and All-cause mortality: A meta-analysis *American Journal of Epidemiology*, Volume 179, Issue 3, 1 February 2014, Pages 282–289, https://doi.org/10.1093/aje/kwt261
3. Demark-Wahnefried W, Price DT, Polascik TJ, et al. Pilot study of dietary fat restriction and flaxseed supplementation in men with prostate cancer before surgery: exploring the effects on hormonal levels, prostate-specific antigen, and histopathologic features. Urology. 2001;58(1):47–52
4. Worldwide cancer statistics. *Cancer Research UK* https://www.cancerresearchuk.org/health-professional/cancer-statistics/worldwide-cancer (2015).
5. 58, Savitri A, Bhavanishankar TN, Desikachar HSR. Effect of spices on in vitro gas production by Clostridium perfringens. Food Microbiol. 1986; 3:195–9.
6. 59. Di Stefano M, Miceli E, Gotti S, Missanelli A, Mazzocchi S, Corazza GR. The effect of oral alpha galactosidase on intestinal gas production and gas-related symptoms. Dig Dis Sci. 2007;52(1):78–83
7. 18 Su CC, Lin JG, Li TM, et al. Curcumin-induced apoptosis of human colon cancer colo 205 cells through the production of ROS, Ca2+, and the activation of caspase-3. Anticancer Res. 2006; 26(6B):4379–89.
8. Hanahan, D., and Weinberg, R. A. (2000). "The hallmarks of cancer." *Cell.* 100(1): 57-70. https://doi.org/10.1016/s0092-8674(00)81683-9.
9. Vaux, David (2011/05/01) - 341- 3. In defense of the Somatic Mutation Theory of Cancer, vol 33, DO - 10.1002/bies 201100022 in BioEssays: news and reviews in molecular, cellular and developmental biology
10. Bäckhed F, Roswall J, Peng Y, et al. Dynamics and stabilization of the human gut microbiome during the first year of life. *Cell Host Microbe* 2015; 17(6):690–703.

11. Roy S, Trinchieri G. Microbiota: a key orchestrator of cancer therapy. *Nat Rev Cancer* 2017; 17(5):271–285.

12. Brown, J. R. & Thornton, J. L. Percivali Pott (1714-1788) and Chimney Sweepers' Cancer of the Scrotum. Br. J. Ind. Med. 14, 68–70 (1957).

13. Yamagiwa, K. & Ichikawa, K. Experimental study of the pathogenesis of carcinoma. J. Cancer Res. 27, 123–81 (1918).

14. Takigawa, M., Verma, A. K., Simsiman, R. C. & Boutwell, R. K. Inhibition of mouse skin tumor promotion and of promoter-stimulated epidermal polyamine biosynthesis by alpha Difluoromethylornithine. Carcinogenesis 43, 3732–8 (1983).

15. krankheiten, ***Berlin***, A. ***Hirschwald, 1894***. 3. Hyde, J. N.: On the Influence *of* Light in the Production *of **Cancer** of* the ***Skin***, Am. J.N. Sc. 131:1, 1906. 4

16. Harting, F. H., and W. Hesse. 1979. Der lungenkrebs, die Bergkrankheit in den Schneeberger gruben. Vjschr. Gerichtl. Med. Offentl. Gesundheitswesen 31:102–132,313–337

17. Dietrich, Holger & Golka, Klaus. (2012). Bladder tumors and aromatic amines - Historical milestones from Ludwig Rehn to Wilhelm Hueper. Frontiers in Bioscience (Elite edition). 4. 279-88. 10.2741/E375.

18. Corrigendum to "Inferring the 1985-2014 impact of mobile phone use on selected brain cancer subtypes using Bayesian structural time series and synthetic controls" [Environ. Int. (2016), 97, 100-107]

19. Campbell TC: Nutrition and cancer: an historical perspective. 1. Was a nutritional association acknowledged a century ago? *Nutr Cancer*, 8(1): 1–7, 2017. doi: 10.1080/01635581.2017.1317823

20. *Venturelli S, Leischner C, Helling T, Renner O, Burkard M, Marongiu L. Minerals and cancer: overview of the possible diagnostic value. Cancers (Basel) 2022; 14(5):1256. doi: 10.3390/cancers14051256.*

21. Prasad AS, Halsted JA, Nadimi M. Syndrome of iron deficiency anemia, hepatosplenomegaly, hypogonadism, dwarfism, and geophagia. Am J Med. 1961; 31:532–46

22. *Warburg O. (1956a). On the origin of cancer cells. Science 123, 309–314. 10.1126/science 123.3191.309*

23. *Warburg O. (1956b). On the respiratory impairment in cancer cells. Science 124, 269–270.*

24. Seyfried T. N. (2012a). Cancer as a Metabolic Disease: On the Origin, Management, and Prevention of Cancer. Hoboken, NJ: John Wiley & Sons

25. H. Vainio, E. Heseltine, J. Wilbourn, (1993) Report on an IARC working group meeting on some naturally occurring substances. *Int J Cancer* **53**, 535-537.

26. N. Benkerroum (2019). Retrospective and Prospective Look at Aflatoxin Research and Development from a Practical Standpoint. *Int J Environ Res Public Health* **16**

27. *Vander Heiden MG, DeBerardinis RJ. (2017). Understanding the Intersections between Metabolism and Cancer Biology. Cell. 168(4):657–669.*

28. Coley-Nauts H, McLaren JR (1990) Coley Toxins – the first century. Adv Exp Med Biol: 267:483.

29. Post-diagnosis social networks, lifestyle, and treatment factors in the After Breast Cancer Pooling Project. Kroenke CH, Michael YL, Shu XO, Poole EM, Kwan ML, Nechuta S, Caan BJ, Pierce JP, Chen WY.Psychooncology. 2017 Apr; 26(4):544-552. doi: 10.1002/pon.4059. Epub 2016 Jan 8. PMID: 26749519

30. Reiche EM, Nunes SO, Morimoto HK. Stress, depression, the immune system, and cancer. Lancet Oncol. 2004 Oct; 5(10):617-25. doi: 10.1016/S1470-2045(04)01597-9. PMID: 15465465.

42. Li H, Jia W. Cometabolism of microbes and host: implications for drug metabolism and drug-induced toxicity. *ClinPharmacol Ther* 2013; 94(5):574–581